An Introduction to Bioethics

SECOND EDITION
Revised and Updated

Thomas A. Shannon

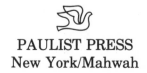

PAULIST PRESS
New York/Mahwah

Library of Congress Cataloging-in-Publication Data

Shannon, Thomas A. (Thomas Anthony), 1940-
    An introduction to bioethics.

    Includes bibliographies.
    1. Medical ethics. 2. Bioethics. I. Title.
[DNLM: 1. Bioethics. 2. Ethics, Medical.
W 50 S528i]
R724.S455   1987   174'.2   87-2377
ISBN 0-8091-2902-7

Published by Paulist Press
997 Macarthur Boulevard
Mahwah, New Jersey 07430

Printed and bound in the
United States of America

Contents

Rededicated
to my brother Jerry and my sister Theresa
with gratitude and thanks for who they are

PREFACE TO
THE REVISED EDITION

When this book was first written seven years ago, I did not realize how popular and widely used it would become—although I certainly had my hopes. As originally published in 1979, the book reached a very broad audience situated in a wide variety of contexts. That was the exact purpose I had in mind.

Although many new developments have occurred and new frontiers have been established, many of the same questions remain and continue to be as perplexing as ever—perhaps even more so given the rapid pace at which developments in medicine continue.

The purpose of the book remains the same: to provide an introduction to general problems in bioethics, to present these problems for a lay audience which seeks to be informed about their ethical dimensions, and to present the basic range of problems and solutions.

Two new chapters have been added: a more thorough discussion of thematic ethical concepts and a chapter on environmental ethics. Other chapters have been updated with respect to new dimensions of the problems. The framing of the issues remains rather constant.

Thomas A. Shannon
Professor of Social Ethics
Department of Humanities
Worcester Polytechnic Institute

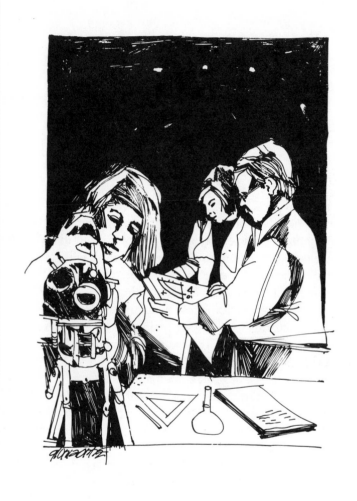

Chapter One

WHAT IS BIOETHICS?

In 1987, the word bioethics has become a commonplace. Several news magazines have devoted special issues to topics such as organ transplants, in vitro fertilization, and the artificial heart. Almost daily, media attention is focused on some particular problem, application, or breakthrough in science that inevitably raises as many problems as the ones it solves.

We have become so used to these discussions and events that we forget it was only twenty-two years ago that the Institute for the Study of Society, Ethics and the Life Sciences—as the Hastings Center was known then—was founded. In 1965, few knew of the Institute—and fewer still knew what they were talking about. But the role and value of this Institute and others that were to follow in its footsteps were soon discovered as the major questions of abortion, population control, the allocation of resources, genetic engineering, behavior modification, and all the problems associated with dying began to press in upon us. Discoveries and applications began to outpace our ability to reflect on them, and everyone was reeling from the biological revolution.

We have seen three Presidential Commissions, an encyclopedia, numerous journals and books, several professional societies, and innumerable conferences all devoted to various problems in bioethics. Courses have spread throughout undergraduate and graduate schools. Ethicists have appeared as experts in court trials. Committees to review the ethical dimensions of human research are present almost everywhere. Similar committees are being proposed to review the cases of dying patients and newborns with birth anomalies.

Few would have thought such events could have happened when the first, few tentative steps were being taken in the early 1960s. From these early days, a wealth of scholarship has been generated, and while many problems seem as intractable as they did when first considered, the field has advanced considerably and we are the beneficiaries of such scholarship.

Since bioethics examines the ethical dimension of problems at the cutting edge of technology, medicine, and biology in their application to life, the area covered is necessarily broad. This is what makes bioethics as a discipline complex but also exciting. It means that a revolution in thinking is called for. Because no one field can claim the territory of life, many specialties and disciplines are needed. Bioethics is teaching us the necessity of genuine interdisciplinary thinking and working. We have learned that medical technologies have economic consequences which raise questions of allocation. Reality—which is interdisciplinary—has taught us to be interdisciplinary in our thinking.

*Bio*ethics

When we focus on the first half of the topic of this book—the "bio" half—we are thrust into the exciting, complex and often troublesome world of medicine, the life sciences, psychology, biotechnology, and genetics. This half of our topic requires that we study these fields to understand the biological revolution that is occurring around us. While we need not be experts, nor even competent amateurs, we do need to be informed citizens if for no other reason than that the developments in these fields have a profound impact on our lives. Thus paying attention to developments in these fields is a critical first step in examining ethical dilemmas in bioethics.

Bio*ethics*

The other half of our topic is equally important, for the developments we have discussed raise serious and profound dilemmas which challenge our value system as well as the culture which is supported by those values.

Ethics, of course, has a problematic reputation. Many regard ethics as the great "nay-sayer" and dismiss it out of hand. Others reduce ethical arguments to opinion or taste and refuse to face arguments and conflicts. Still others use carefully developed methodologies to consider various values and to tease out hidden conflicts and complex relationships.

Let me present an overview of two methods of ethical decision making which are frequently used in bioethics. The first goes by the imposing name of deontological ethics. The Greek word "deon" means duty, obligation, or principle. Deontological ethics is a method of decision making which begins by asking "What are my duties?" or "What are my obligations?" The correct ethical course is to follow one's principles—regardless of where they lead. I frequently refer to this as the "Damn the torpedoes, full steam ahead" school of ethics. For once duties or obligations are established, the appropriate actions are clear.

A very commonplace example of deontological or principle-based ethics is the ten commandments of the Judaeo-Christian tradition. The ten commandments are basically a set of moral duties that tell what to do and what not to do. They are presented as clear and certain moral guides that mean what they say and say what they mean.

A second approach is called consequentalism. This is because moral obligations are established not by an evaluation of obligations, but by an examination of consequences. Thus the name consequentalism. This method attempts to predict what will happen if one acts in various ways and to compare the outcomes against each other. What is moral or the right act is determined through the evaluative process.

Situation ethics is probably the best known of the many variants of consequentalism. Popularized in the mid 1960s by

Joseph Fletcher, situation ethics requires that we attend seriously to the implications of actualizing our ethical beliefs. Thus consequentalism would argue that it is not enough to do good; one must also know which of the many possible goods is best.

The Issues

The issues or topics to be discussed in this introduction are the table of contents, which presents only the generic listing of topics. Thus the book will present an overview of the issues in the major problem areas of bioethics: technology, abortion, death and dying, newborns with birth anomalies, organ transplantation, research on human subjects, behavior modification, genetic engineering, patients' rights, and environmental issues.

As you proceed into the book, you will notice that certain questions continue to reappear, certain terms continue to make their significance felt. Certain questions and solutions to problems will raise broader social policy questions. Fundamental relationships and values are called into question by certain practices. This introduction will not examine these topics or subjects, but will frame various questions so that you will have a way of orienting yourself to these broader questions of social policy.[1]

In 1977 the philosopher Samuel Gorovitz defined bioethics as the "critical examination of the moral dimensions of decision-making in health-related contexts and in contexts involving the biological sciences."[2] This definition is still a good one, for it highlights the interdisciplinary and social dimensions of bioethics. It points us in the right direction as we enter the fascinating, but complex world of bioethics.

Notes

1. For an in-depth examination of these and other topics, I suggest my reader entitled *Bioethics: Selected Readings* which is also available in a revised edition from Paulist Press. The

reader presents articles which cover a broad range of perspectives for each of the topics covered here in outline fashion.

2. Samuel Gorovitz, "Bioethics and Social Responsibility," *The Monist* 60 (January 1977) 3.

Discussion Questions

1. Why is it necessary to have basic knowledge of both scientific and ethical issues in considering the problems encountered in bioethics?

2. What major bioethical problems have been in the media recently? What are some of their implications?

3. Why must one also consider the social or policy implications of problems in bioethics?

Bibliography

Tom L. Beauchamp and LeRoy Walters, editors, *Contemporary Issues in Bioethics*. Dickinson Publishing Company, 1978.

Joseph Fletcher, *Morals and Medicine*. Beacon Press, 1954.

———, *Humanhood. Essays in Biomedical Ethics*. Prometheus Books, 1979.

Samuel Gorovitz et al., editors, *Moral Problems in Medicine*. Prentice-Hall, 1976.

Frank Harron et al., *Health and Human Values. A Guide to Making Your Own Decisions*. Yale University Press, 1983.

Immanuel Jakobovitz, *Jewish Medical Ethics*. Block Publishing Co., 1959.

David Kelly, *The Emergence of Roman Catholic Medical Ethics in North America*. The Edwin Mellen Press, 1979.

Gerard Kelly, *Medico-Moral Problems*. The Catholic Hospital Association, 1958.

Carol Levine, editor, *Taking Sides: Clashing Values on Controversial Bioethical Issues*. The Dushkin Publishing Group, 1984.

William F. May, *The Physician's Covenant. Images of the Healer in Medical Ethics*. The Westminster Press, 1983.

Richard McCormick, *How Brave a New World?* Georgetown University Press, 1981.

Paul Ramsey, *The Patient as Person*. Yale University Press, 1970.

——, *Ethics at the Edges of Life: Medical and Legal Perspectives*. Yale University Press, 1978.

Warren Reich, general editor, *The Encyclopedia of Bioethics,* 4 vols. The Free Press, 1978.

Thomas A. Shannon, *Bioethics: Selected Readings*. Paulist Press, Revised Edition, 1981.

Thomas A. Shannon and Joann Manfra, editors, *Law and Bioethics*. Paulist Press, 1982.

Nadya Shmavonian, *Human Values in Medicine and Health Care: Audio-Visual Resources*. The Vail-Ballou Press, 1983. This work lists 400 A-V resources and is a helpful resource.

Paul Starr, *The Social Transformation of American Medicine*. Basic Books, 1982.

Robert M. Veatch, *Case Studies in Bioethics*. Harvard University Press, 1977.

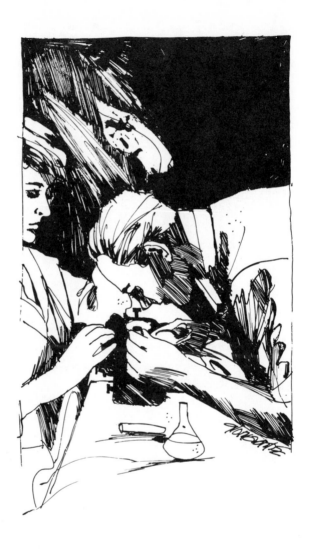

Chapter Two

THE ROLE AND
PLACE OF TECHNOLOGY

Introduction

Humans have always seemed to find ways of intervening in nature. The ability to make a fire and the invention of the wheel had profound impacts on the development of human society. The domestication of plants and animals allowed humans to live in ways unthought of before. The rise of modern science and the Industrial Revolution stand as markers of yet another major change in our way of life.

Our current technological revolution presents further opportunities and capacities for intervening in life on both the micro and macro levels. The technologies surrounding conception and birth, such as in vitro fertilization and amniocentesis, help determine when we will be born and what some of our qualities may (or may not) be. Developments in genetics led to the production of new grains that produce more bushels per acre. An oil eating bacterium has been manufactured to help clean up oil spills. And the artificial heart is now a reality.

Hardly an area of our lives is not touched by technology. But the record of technology is certainly a mixed one. Clearly technology has brought benefits. Computers have given us incredible capacities for calculating and information processing. Medical technologies provide improved diagnostic capacities.

Other technologies have fairly negative consequences. Nuclear weapons have brought us to the brink of annihilation. More sophisticated instruments of "interrogation" continue to be developed. The impact of yet other technologies is mixed. Nuclear power stations provide necessary energy but problems of waste disposal have yet to be satisfactorily resolved. Birth technologies provide children, but are such children reduced to commodities?

Whatever one's judgment about a particular technology, technology is here to stay and will continue to have far-reaching effects on our lives.

Characteristics of Technology

While technologies vary, technology has several common themes. Let me indicate several of these by following some ideas proposed by Norman Faramelli in his book *Technethics*.[1]

a. The empirical or pragmatic spirit. This is certainly close to the American spirit. We want to get the job done and done quickly. The issue is results, preferably results that we can measure.

b. Functionalism. Functionalism follows from the pragmatic bent of our culture. The issue is design and performance. We are frequently more concerned about how something will work than why we should do it.

c. Preoccupation with means, not ends. We know that it is often easier to figure out how to solve a particular problem than to agree on which problem ought to be solved. The question of ends requires explicit value judgments for solutions. We often hope that we can finesse that difficult debate by focusing on the means—and by pretending that the means debate involves no value or ethical judgments.

d. Preference for quantity over quality. An old song has it that if you can't be with the one you love, then love the one you're with. This attitude reflects—among other things—a preference for that which is at hand, for what is available, rather than that which is better. Of course, quantitative measurements are easier to do and the phrase "the bottom line" has a nice objective, realistic ring to it. Yet for all the material goods available to us, we seem so unsatisfied, unfulfilled.

e. Efficiency and profit. The concept of standardization led to the development of interchangeable parts which led to mass production which led to fewer skilled laborers being needed which led to lower wages which led to higher profits. Pragmatism, functionalism, and preoccupation with means and quantity all join here to promote efficiency in the service of higher profits.

f. Manipulation. Concern for efficiency and quantity lead to a desire to exercise greater rational control over all phases of life. For only in this way can productivity be increased at a cost-effective level. Manipulation to achieve rational control is one thread in the manufacturing process—though the final word on the use of robots is yet to be heard. But such manipulation may be quite another thing when we begin mass-producing people.

What Is Technology?

Having seen some of the characteristics of technology, let's now look to define it. An obvious approach to technology is through hardware—the machines, the instruments, the robots. This is certainly an important part of technology, for this dimension of it clearly has a major impact on our lives.

Others, however, like Jacques Ellul—a French theologian—see technology more as technique.[2] Technique is a complex of standardized means for achieving a pre-determined result. This result is obtained through a deliberate and rationalized process, using many of the characteristics of technology described above. Technique is the rational organization of behavior, not hardware or output.

This orientation is more helpful because it allows us to see technology as a cultural phenomenon, a method of organization, an angle of vision. While the products of the technological revolution impact our lives, our social reality is affected more profoundly by technology as an organizational method for both thought and social interaction.

Daniel Bell of Harvard University has also analyzed technology and has defined five essential dimensions: function, energy, fabrication, communication and control, and regulated decision making.[3]

a. Function. Function is the primary element in design and is related to nature only insofar as nature is an efficient guide. As noted before, the issue is how something performs, not why we need to have this done.

b. Energy. The technological revolution gradually demanded new power sources, and that need was fulfilled by shifting from natural sources such as wind, water, and personal strength to manufactured sources such as steam and electricity. Now that the natural resources required for their generation are becoming depleted, we are turning to nuclear power. Our need for power is outstripping our capacity to generate it, and this is creating a crisis, nationally and internationally.

c. Fabrication. Bell uses this word to describe the process of standardization of both parts and actions. This permits the replacement of one part or person with another so that greater efficiency can be achieved. One can use this process in manufacturing, in organizing a corporation, or in education.

d. Communication and control. Technological systems feed off information and require increasing amounts of it to keep the system going. Thus, whoever controls the communication system controls the power. Information is useless unless it is communicated, and technology, through increasing utilization of computer networks, provides an increasingly effective and efficient method of communication and control.

e. Decision-making rules. Since function, fabrication, and communication are critical parts of the technological culture, we need to be assured that there will be coherence in their use and application. Rules of communication and decision-making cannot be random or spontaneous, or the vital flow of information may be interrupted. Thus there is a need for speed and accuracy in the decision-making process which calls for greater standardization. This, of course, leads to a greater centralization of power and reinforces communication and control systems.

But whether understood as hardware or a mode of thought or a system, technology has profound effects on our everyday lives. Because of this, people see the need to examine technology to predict its effects and to evaluate them. Such assessments will, we hope, help us avoid many undesirable consequences of a particular technology.

One such method of evaluation is the technological assessment. This is a systematic study of the effects on society that may occur when a technology is introduced, expanded, or modified, with special emphasis on the impacts that are unintended, indirect, and delayed. It attempts to evaluate a broad range of effects including, but not limited to, environmental, social, economic, and political. Thus, a technological assessment seeks to examine as thoroughly as possible, the short and long term consequences of a technology, its risks and benefits, its social and environmental impacts, and the cultural implications. Only by attending to all of these dimensions can one obtain a full sense of the significance of a technology.

Types of Technology

In his study of technology, Daniel Callahan identified five types of technology.[4] The purpose of developing this classification schema was to help us see the potential of various technologies as well as understand the impact various technologies have on our lives.

a. Preservation technologies. These technologies help us adapt to nature or to survive various environments so that we can fit into our environment, or help us investigate our environment. Some examples of these technologies are our homes, furnaces, irrigation systems, eyeglasses, and telescopes.

b. Improvement technologies. Technologies such as these enable people to meet their felt needs or to go beyond the limits of their particular natural capabilities. As such, improvement technologies can enhance our physical dimensions or can help decorate or embellish our bodies. Examples of these are genetic engineering, prosthetics, and cosmetic surgery.

c. Implementation technologies. These technologies are difficult to describe because their purpose is to assist in the implementation of other technologies. One can best think of these technologies as facilitators or enhancers. Thus the computer allows us access to other information technologies and the telephone allows us access to information. Planned obsolescence or the changing fashion allows people to have work.

d. Destructive technologies. Technologies such as these are designed with one primary purpose: destruction. They may help us achieve other ends, but the purpose of these technologies is clear from their design. Such technologies may achieve their end through manipulation and control or simply by the capacity for obliteration. Examples are behavior modification technologies, weapon systems and vacuum aspirators.

e. Compensatory technologies. Having developed and implemented all manner of technologies, we now need other technologies to help us deal with the effects of these technologies on our lives. Thus we have machines to help us exercise, we have music to help drown out the noise of technology, and we have sensitivity training to enable us to experience the world we have removed through technology.

Summary

If we look around us, it is clear that technology is here to stay. Our culture is utterly dependent on various aspects of it.

We could not get through our day without technology. From clocks to microwaves to transportation systems to VCRs, our lives, work and entertainment are inherently tied up with technology.

Our quality of life has greatly increased because of technology. We live in greater comfort in various climates. We have abundant food and water supplies, we can communicate and travel much more efficiently, and our health has improved.

But we also suffer from the terrors of technology. We stand in daily dread of the release of weapons that would destroy us. We have more information accessible to us but we know less of what it means or what to do with it. Pollution, a by-product of our technical culture, is threatening to destroy our ecosystem.

Thus many benefits and problems are given to us by technology. Each requires study and examination. But it is to one application of technology—the medical—that we now turn for further examination.

Notes

1. Norman J. Faramelli, *Technethics*. Friendship Press, 1971, p. 31ff.

2. Jacques Ellul, *The Technological Society*. Vintage Books, 1964, pp. 13ff.

3. Daniel Bell, Faculty Seminar Presentation, Worcester Polytechnic Institute, 1976. Confer also *The Coming of the Post-Industrial Society*. Basic Books, 1975.

4. Daniel Callahan, *The Tyranny of Survival*. Macmillan, 1973, pp. 55ff.

Topics for Discussion

1. What are the costs and benefits, the strengths and weaknesses of the vast technological society that has developed in America?

2. What are some examples of unintended and delayed side-effects of technology? Do you think these could have been avoided?

3. Develop lists of examples of the various types of technologies. What needs are these technologies meant to satisfy? What values are these technologies based on?

4. How has technology benefited your life? How has it complicated your life?

5. Which is more helpful for you: to think of technology as hardware or as a system? Why?

Bibliography

Ian Barbour, editor, *Science and Religion*. Harper and Row, 1968.

Daniel Bell, *The Coming of the Post-Industrial Society*. Basic Books, 1973.

Joseph Bronowsky, *Science and Human Values*. Harper and Row, 1965.

Daniel Callahan, *The Tyranny of Survival*. Macmillan, 1973.

Jacques Ellul, *The Technological Society*. Vintage Books, 1964.

Victor C. Ferkiss, *The Failure of Technological Civilization*. George Braziller, 1974.

———, *Technological Man: The Myth and the Reality*. George Braziller, 1969.

Garrett Hardin, *Exploring New Ethics For Survival: The Voyage of Spaceship Beagle*. Viking Press, 1972.

Thomas Kuhn, *The Structure of Scientific Revolutions*. University of Chicago Press, 1970.

Marc Lappe, *Genetic Politics: The Limits of Biological Control*. Simon and Schuster, 1977.

Donald MacKay, *Human Science and Human Dignity*. Intervarsity Press, 1979.

Roger Shinn, *Forced Options. Social Decisions for the 21st Century*. Harper and Row, 1982.

Roger Shinn and Paul Abrecht, editors, *Faith and Science in an Unjust World*. Report of the World Council of Churches' Conference on Faith, Science, and the Future, 2 vols. The World Council of Churches, 1981.

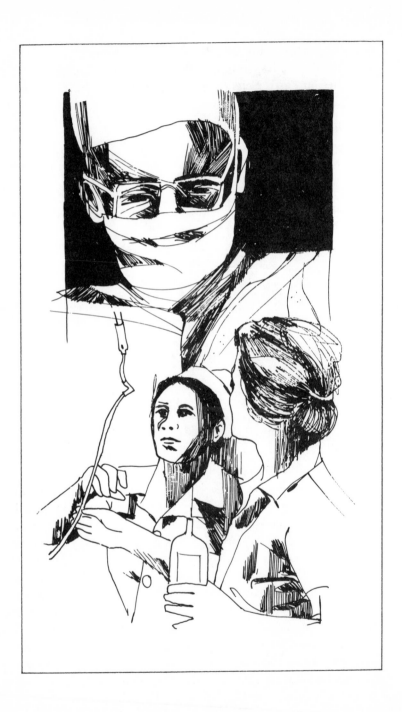

Chapter Three

ETHICAL ISSUES

To prepare you for some of the discussions that will emerge in the various topics and help give you a basic framework for ethical analysis, this chapter will present, first, a discussion of ethical theories or methods and, second, definitions of basic ethical concepts.

Ethical Theories

In general, an ethical theory is the process by which we justify a particular ethical decision. It is a means by which we organize complex information and competing values and interests and formulate an answer to the question "What should I do?" The main purpose of a theory is to provide consistency and coherence in our decision-making. That is, an ethical theory or framework gives us a common means to approach various problems. If we have a theory, we don't have to figure out where to begin each time we meet a new problem. A theory also allows us to develop some degree of consistency in our decision-making. We will begin to see how different values relate to each other. If we are consistent and coherent in our decision-making, we will have a greater degree of internal unity and integrity in our decision-making. Given the complexity of problems to be addressed, these qualities are extremely worthwhile.

Consequentialism

The ethical theory of consequentialism answers the question "What should I do?" by considering the consequences of various answers. That is, what is ethical is that consequence which brings about the greatest number of advantages over disadvantages or which brings about the greatest good for the greatest number of people. Basically, in this method, one looks to outcomes, to consequences, to the situation, and, from that perspective, one decides what is ethical. The ethical theories of situation ethics and utilitarianism are frequently used types of consequentialist ethical theories.

The major benefit of this theory is that it looks to the actual impact of a particular decision and asks how people will be affected by it. Consequentialism is attuned to the nuances of life and seeks to be responsive to them. The major problem of this theory is that the theory itself provides no standard by which one would measure one outcome against another. That is, while being sensitive to the circumstances, consequentialism has no basis for evaluating one outcome against another.

Deontologism

Deontological ethics, which derives its name from the Greek word for duty, "deon," looks to one's obligations to determine what is ethical. This theory answers the question "What should I do?" by specifying my obligations or moral duties. That is, the ethical act is one in which I meet my obligations, my responsibilities, or fulfill my duties. For a deontologist, obligation and rules are primary, for only by attending to these dimensions of morality can one be sure that self-interest does not override moral obligations. The ten commandments and Kant's categorical imperative are probably the most common examples of deontological ethics.

The major benefit of deontological ethics is the clarity and certainty of its starting point. Once the rules are known or the duties determined, then what is ethical is evident. The major problem is the potential insensitivity to consequences. By looking only at duty, one may miss important aspects of a problem.

Rights Ethics

This theory resolves ethical dilemmas by first determining what rights or moral claims are involved. Then dilemmas are resolved in terms of the hierarchy of rights. Paramount for a person of this orientation is that the moral claims of individuals—their rights—are taken seriously. The ethical theory of rights is a popular one in our American culture. Consider, for example, the central role that this theory plays in the abortion debate.

The main advantage of a rights theory is that it highlights the moral centrality of the person and his or her moral claims in a situation of ethical conflict. On the other hand, this theory does not tell us how to resolve conflicts of rights between individuals. The theory makes the claims of the individual central without telling us how to resolve potential conflicts of rights.

Intuitionism

Intuitionism resolves ethical dilemmas by appealing to one's intuition, a moral faculty of the person which directly apprehends what is right or wrong. Thus an intuitionist knows what is right or wrong, not by appeal to circumstances, duties, or rights, but by appeal to one's moral sense. While one's intuition may confer duties, the duty is not the point of departure; one's moral sense is.

We all know of situations in which all we can say is, "I'm doing this because I know it's right," and that is the end of the moral argument. Experientially we know that we frequently rely on this method, and the strength that comes from such a moral intuition is great. Nonetheless, if we cannot externalize or publicize in some fashion our process of decision-making, we cannot be totally accountable to others. Thus while intuitionism may give us the necessary courage of our convictions, it does not provide us with a way of convincing others that our way is correct.

Summary

As you read this book and discuss the problems contained in it, you will find yourself using one or more of these methods in trying to convince yourself or others of the correctness of a particular position. You may also find it interesting to adopt one method to see how it works and where it will lead you. Discovering which method you are more comfortable with and being attentive to the methods others are using is a first step toward gaining clarity in one's discussions and debates about complex medical-ethical dilemmas.

Ethical Terms

In the course of this book various terms will be frequently used. Philosophers, like physicians, nurses, lawyers, and other professionals, have their own language and jargon. This section will introduce you to some of the basic terms used in bioethical discussions so you can join in on the conversations.

Autonomy

Autonomy is a form of personal liberty of action in which the individual determines his or her course of action in accordance with a plan of his or her own choosing. Autonomy involves two elements. First is the capacity to deliberate about a plan of action. One must be capable of examining alternatives and distinguishing between them. Second, one must have the capacity to put one's plan into action. Autonomy includes the ability to actualize or carry out what one has decided.

In many ways, autonomy is the all-American value or virtue. It affirms that we ought to be the master of our own fate or the captain of our ship. Autonomy mandates a strong sense of personal responsibility for our own lives. Autonomy celebrates the hardy individualism for which our country is famous. It emphasizes creativity and productivity while being the enemy of conformity. Autonomy mandates that we choose who we wish to be and take responsibility for that.

In celebrating individuality and control of one's self, too heavy a reliance on autonomy can isolate one from the community, from one's family, from one's friends. While ultimately I am responsible for myself and my actions, the community can also be involved in my learning what my responsibilities are and can also set obligations that I need to respect as I make my decisions.

Thus, while autonomy is important, and plays a critical role in bioethics, it needs to be understood within the context of the community as well as other moral responsibilities that I may have.[1]

Nonmaleficence

Nonmaleficence is the technical way of stating that we have an obligation not to harm people, one of the most traditional ethical principles of medical ethics. "First of all, do no harm." This is the basic principle derived from the Hippocratic tradition. If we can't benefit someone, then at least we should do that person no harm.

The harm we are to avoid is typically understood as physical or mental. But harm can also include injuries to one's interests. Thus I can be harmed by having my property unjustly taken or by having my access to it restricted. Or I can be harmed by having my liberty of speech or action unfairly restricted. Although there is no necessary physical impact on me from these latter harms, nonetheless I am harmed by having my interests constrained.

The duty of nonmaleficence clearly imposes an obligation not to harm someone intentionally or directly. However, it is also possible to expose others to a risk of harm. For example, if I am driving too fast, I may not actually harm someone, but I am clearly exposing individuals to the risk of harm. Thus the duty of nonmaleficence would prohibit speeding.[2]

But there are other situations in which individuals are exposed to the risk of harm, and the duty of nonmaleficence is not necessarily violated. An individual receiving chemotherapy is exposed to various risks of harm from the therapy. Can such risks of harm be justified and, if so, how?

The traditional method for examining the legitimation of risks or harmful effects is the principle of double effect. This tradition has its origin in traditional Roman Catholic theology but has gained wide acceptance as a means of judging the moral acceptability of risks and harms.

The principle of double effect[3] has four conditions:

1. What we are going to do must not be evil or wrong. This is simply a restatement of the traditional moral axiom that we are never allowed to do wrong.

2. The harm we are considering must not be the means of producing the good effect. Our proposed action has a harmful dimension but the good end does not justify the means. We cannot do something wrong simply because a good consequence may also follow.

3. The evil or harmful effect may not be intended, but merely permitted or tolerated. For example, when someone has cardiac bypass surgery, one undergoes a risk of death; one suffers the direct physical harm of having one's rib cage split open. However, the purpose of the operation is to repair blocked heart arteries, not to cut open one's chest. To repair the arteries, the chest must be cut open.

4. There must be a proportionate reason for performing the action in spite of the consequences the act has. This requires us to weigh a variety of benefits and costs, of values and disvalues. In doing this, one should ensure that the good outweighs the bad. Otherwise the second condition is violated.

In making this proportionalist judgment, Richard McCormick[4] has identified three factors to take into consideration. First, there is at stake a value at least equal in importance to the one sacrificed. Second, there is no less harmful way, here and now, of protecting the good we are seeking to attain. Third, the way that the value is achieved should not undermine that value in the future.

McCormick's point is that establishing a proportionate reason is not like solving an arithmetic problem. Rather we need to exercise prudence and gauge the effect of our acts on other values. The duty of nonmaleficence stands as a strong reminder that we have an obligation not to harm, but that when some harm or risk of harm appears to be necessary, then we need to be accountable. The principle of double effect provides that process of justification.

Beneficence

Beneficence is the positive dimension of nonmaleficence. The duty of beneficence claims that we have a duty to help others further their interests when we can do this without risk to ourselves. Thus the duty of beneficence argues that we have a positive obligation to regard the welfare of others, to be of assistance to others as they attempt to fulfill their plans. The duty of beneficence is based on a sense of fair play. It basically suggests that because we have received benefits from others, because we have been helped along the way, we have an obligation to return that same favor to others. Beneficence is a way of ensuring reciprocity in our relations and of passing along to others the goods we have received in the past.[5]

But this duty is not without limit. The limit is harm to oneself. Beauchamp and Childress have identified a process which one can use to evaluate the risk of harm to determine our degree of obligation. First, the individual we are to help is at risk of significant loss or danger. Second, I can perform an act directly relevant to preventing this loss or damage. Third, my act is likely to prevent this damage or loss. Fourth, the benefits that the individual receives as a consequence of my actions (a) outweigh harms to self and (b) present minimal risk to self.[6]

Again we have the necessity of making a prudential calculation about risks and benefits. Sometimes this calculation may be clear. If someone is drowning and I cannot swim, I am not obligated to go in the water to help the person, although I would be obligated to assist in other ways. But the calculation may be problematic. Does a health care professional have a duty to care for someone with AIDS? Here the moral calculus is complicated because of unclarity about the method of transmission, the time of incubation, and the effectiveness of traditional isolation techniques, as well as the as yet incurable nature of the disease.

Justice

On the one hand, the basic meaning or intent of justice is rather straightforward. Justice deals with the allocation of resources. It is the distribution of benefits and burdens, of goods and services according to a just standard. But determining that just standard has perplexed and puzzled people down through the ages.[7]

There are two basic types of justice. Comparative justice argues that what one person or group receives is determined by balancing the competing claims of other individuals or groups. In comparative justice, what one receives is determined by one's conditions or needs and how those relate to similar needs of others in society. Thus one person may need a kidney transplant more than another because person A is dying of renal failure while person B has just been diagnosed as having kidney disease. The point of comparative justice is a balancing of the needs of individuals competing for the same resource.

Noncomparative justice determines distribution of goods or resources by a standard independent of the claims of others. Here we have a principle of distribution or treatment, not an evaluation of the specifics of the case or the needs of the individuals. Good examples of noncomparative standards are the distribution according to strict numerical equality or the legal rule that all are innocent until proven guilty. In noncomparative justice, allocation, distribution or treatment is determined by principle, not need.

Similarly, there are two basic principles of justice: formal and material. The formal principle of justice specifies a procedure to be followed in allocating goods or distributing burdens. The traditional principle of justice is derivative from the Greek philosopher Aristotle: equals are to be treated equally and unequals unequally—or, to restate it, to each his or her own.

The formal principle of justice is noncomparative in that it states a rule by which distributions are to be measured. It proposes a standard independent of needs or individuals. However, the rule does not tell how we determine what qualifies for equality or inequality. That is, with respect to what standard is someone equal or unequal? What is morally relevant in our determining equality or inequality? The strength of the formal principle of justice is that it gives us a clear rule; its major deficit is that it does not specify how to apply it.

To cope with the problem of applications, material principles of justice have been devised. Generally speaking, a material principle of justice identifies some relevant property or criterion on the basis of which a distribution can be made. Thus material principles of justice are typically, though not always, comparative in that they examine needs or qualifications and on that basis determine what to do. Let me illustrate this by identifying several of these material principles of justice.

First is the noncomparative material principle of to each an equal share. The standard is strict numerical equality, and one arrives at this by dividing what is to be allocated by the number of actual recipients. Second is distribution according to individual need. Here one looks at specific needs of individuals and judges them, one against the other. This, like the third principle of justice—social worth—is obviously comparative. Social worth criteria go beyond needs and evaluate the status of an individual or his or her actual or potential contributions to society. The final form of material justice, which is also comparative, is distribution according to individual effort. This criterion does not examine accomplishments but looks at what one attempted and the efforts to realize that. The higher the effort, the greater the reward.

Each of these principles has its benefits and problems, and because of this a middle way has been suggested. This method of allocation emphasizes formal equality but shifts this by utilizing equality of opportunity rather than one of the comparative forms of justice. This method of distribution is randomization either through a lottery or by distribution to people as they show up.

The obvious benefit of this method is that it protects

strongly our intuitive sense of respect for people. That is, randomization provides a formal rule of allocation that does not force us to make invidious and potentially harmful choices between people based on assumptions about social worth. Individuals maintain their dignity because they will be treated fairly by having an equality of opportunity. Finally, such a system will help maintain trust between members of the health care team and the patient. The patient is not at the mercy of biases of an institution or individuals, but rather knows that he or she will be treated fairly.

On the other hand, this standard does not deal with some important questions. First, should there be some medical screen through which one should pass before entering the door? Second, should one's condition or likelihood of benefit be considered? That is, if a fifteen year old is more likely to benefit from a procedure than an eighty year old, should the eighty year old have an equal opportunity for treatment? Third, the mode of distribution assumes an endless supply of resources in that the only relevant criterion is equality of opportunity, not appropriateness of intervention or resource allocation.

From this discussion one can easily see why discussions of justice are important in bioethics, but also why they are among the most complex.

Informed Consent

Informed consent is, I think, the most critical problem in bioethics. This is the time when health care professionals and patients can discuss value implications of treatments or clarify what is important for each of them. Consent negotiations allow discussions of issues of importance for all involved parties.

Informed consent is the knowledge of and consent to a particular form of treatment before that treatment is administered. In this definition are four major elements.[8]

1. Competence. Competence generally refers to a person's capacity for decision-making. A person may experience full competence, in that he or she is in control of one's life. Or competence may be limited. A person may have decision-making capacities in one area but not another. An individual may not comprehend the value of money and may be restrained in its use but may be quite capable of making other decisions of daily living concerning nutrition, personal hygiene, or appointment-making. Age may also limit competence in that one may be competent for some activities but not others. Finally, and most difficult, one may be intermittently competent. Consider, for example, persons becoming senile. At times these individuals may be competent, but at other times they may be unaware of the implications of their choices.

To help sort out the difficult issues of evaluating competence, three different standards have been proposed. I will present them in order of increasing complexity. The first standard states that a person is competent when he or she has made a decision. When presented with a choice, the individual chooses an alternative. The fact of a choice is evidence of competence. Second is the capacity to give reasons for one's choice. Competence here requires some process of justification, an articulation of why one made this choice. The third standard argues that not only should one be able to give reasons for one's choice, but also that this choice should be a reasonable one.

Each of these standards is different and raises a variety of value judgments. What is most critical is that individuals be aware of what standard of competence they are using and recognize that it may conflict with the judgment of others.

2. Disclosure. Disclosure refers to the content of what a patient is told during the consent negotiation. Two general standards for disclosure have been proposed. The first and more traditional standard is the professional standard. What a person is told is what professionals typically tell patients. The obligation to inform patients is fulfilled by telling a patient what one's colleagues would tell that same patient. The obvious problem with this standard is that one's colleagues may tell a patient little or nothing. That is, the professional standard may be simply to tell a patient as little as possible about one's condition.

In this situation, the standard is met, the obligation is fulfilled, but the patient remains ignorant.

Obvious problems with that standard led to the development of the more recent standard of the reasonable person. In this perspective, the health care provider is obligated to disclose what the reasonable person would want to know. One cannot fulfill the obligation by saying nothing; some information must be communicated. And the degree of specificity is centered outside the profession in the hypothetical reasonable person. Such a standard promotes autonomy and is protective of patients' rights. Nonetheless it remains on a general level.

This level of generality is why I think it important to go further and determine what *this particular* patient wants to know. Such a standard of disclosure recognizes a patient's right to be informed but, more importantly, it mediates that right with respect to the patient's desires. Some patients may want to know nothing; others may want additional reading they can do. Only by determining what this particular patient wants to know can his or her rights be respected and protected.

3. Comprehension. In addition to having information disclosed, one must also comprehend that information. If a patient doesn't understand what he or she has been told, there is no way that individual can use the information.

Comprehension presents many problems and may test the patience of health care professionals. Some may assume that patients simply cannot understand the complexity of the issues. Others may assume that one does not comprehend unless one receives a mini-course in medicine. Or one may assume that there is not sufficient time to fully inform an individual.

Several issues should be noted here. First, from the fact that someone is not *fully* informed, it does not follow that he or she is not *adequately* informed. Second, health care professionals have a professional language. While that language is appropriate for peer communication, it is inappropriate for communication with patients. Thus, professionals need to translate their terms and jargon so that it will be intelligible to others. Third, comprehension typically requires time, especially when what needs to be told is not good news. Being informed does not necessitate being told everything at once. Fulfilling the condition of comprehension requires a sensitivity to what a patient can take in at one time.

4. Voluntariness. Voluntariness refers to one's ability to make a choice without being unduly pressured to make a particular choice by any specific person. Being free in making a decision means that we own the decision, that the decision is ours, that we have chosen the option.

It seems clear to me that no decision is ever made without some contraints or pressures. No one chooses in a vacuum, in the absence of values or experiences. The moral issue is to remove as much coercion or undue influence as possible so that the decision is the individual's, not someone else's.

Coercion refers to the use of an actual threat of harm or some type of forceful manipulation to influence the person to choose one alternative rather than another. Coercion may take physical, psychological or economic forms. The nature of coercion is perhaps best captured in the widely quoted phrase from the move *The Godfather:* "I made him an offer he couldn't refuse." This connotes the illusion of choice (made an offer) but, in effect, forecloses all options but one (the one that can't be refused).

Undue influence refers to the use of excessive rewards or irrationally persuasive techniques to short-circuit a person's decision-making process. Thus one may use behavior modification techniques to get someone to agree with your decision. One may offer large cash payments or the promise of benefits to induce people to participate in research that has a high risk.

But in either case, the appeal is not to a person's interests, rights, or values. The purpose of coercion or undue influence is to do an end run around choice or judgment so that the patient will do what he or she might not ordinarily have done.

Paternalism

Generally speaking, paternalism involves some sort of interference with the individual's liberty of action. Typically this interference is justified with reference to the person's own good. Paternalism may be *active* in that one acts on behalf of a person but not at his or her request. One may provide a therapy for a person that the person has not asked for. Or paternalism may be *passive* in that one refuses to help another achieve some goal that he or she may have. For example, a physician may refuse to prescribe a tranquilizer because of fears of its abuse by the patient.

James Childress, in his recent book on paternalism,[9] has identified several types that refine this general idea and indicate its different aspects.

1. Pure and Impure. Pure paternalism bases its intervention into a person's life on an appeal to the welfare of that person alone. This is the classic model in which parents tell children to eat spinach because it's good for them. Impure paternalism justifies interference with another person because of the welfare of that person *and* the welfare of another. Thus, some argue that a parent who is also a Jehovah's Witness should have a blood transfusion not only because of the good for that person, but also for the good of his or her children.

2. Restricted and Extended. A restricted paternalistic intervention is one which overrides an individual's act because of some defect in the person. Thus, one may prohibit a child from doing something because of chronological or psychological incompetence. In extended paternalism, an individual is restrained because what he or she wants to do is risky or dangerous. Thus there are laws that mandate wearing helmets while riding motorcycles or seatbelts while in front seats of cars or when under ten years of age.

3. Positive and Negative. A positive paternalistic act, such as forcing a patient into a rehabilitation program, seeks to promote the person's own good. A negative paternalistic intervention, such as taking cigarettes away from someone, seeks to prevent a harm.

4. Soft and Hard. In a soft paternalistic act, the values used to justify the intervention are the patient's values. For example, unconscious or comatose patients are frequently removed from life support systems because they stated that preference in advance of being in that situation. In hard paternalism, the values used to justify an act are not the patient's. This is the classic case of someone else knowing what is good for you and then having you do it or having it done to you.

5. Direct and Indirect. In direct paternalism, the person who receives the alleged benefit is the one whose values are overridden. The motorcyclist forced to wear the helmet is the one who assumedly will benefit if there is an accident. In indirect paternalism, one person is restrained so that another individual can receive a benefit. A classic instance is child abuse in which parents are restrained in some fashion to benefit the child.

The desire to help someone or provide a benefit for someone runs deep within the human spirit. Also there are the specific obligations of nonmaleficence and beneficence that we discussed earlier in this chapter. Yet people are autonomous. They know their interests and what is important to them. Respect for persons mandates a presumption against paternalistic interventions. Yet we see harm being done that could be prevented. Can the issues be resolved?

One argument for a paternalistic intervention included these four steps:

a. The recipient of the paternalistic act actually has some incapacity which prevents or inhibits him or her from making a decision. The person is under undue stress, is a minor, or his or her judgment is impaired in some way.

b. There is the probability of harm unless there is an intervention. Here one needs to determine if all harms are equal. Are physical, mental, or social harms interchangeable?

c. Proportionality. The probable benefit of intervention outweighs the probable risk of harm from nonintervention. Here one needs to be careful of uncritical interventions of extended paternalism.

d. The paternalistic intervention is the least restrictive, least humiliating and least insulting alternative. This criterion argues that one remain as respectful of the individual as possible during the intervention.

This method will not resolve all issues connected with paternalism, but it will force individuals to recognize and justify such paternalistic interventions.[10]

Rights

The term "rights" is one of the most frequently used in ethics and bioethics. Yet the term is problematic because of its varied meanings and different connotations. This problem is evident even in the origin of the term "rights." In the medieval ethical tradition, we do not find the term "rights"; rather, we find the term "duty." The term "duty" referred to the reciprocal obligation that members of a community had to each other. Duties were specific ways in which each helped the other realize the common good of all. In the modern tradition, beginning with the Enlightenment, rights referred to claims of the individual against the state. Rights were a means of carving out a zone of privacy or protection against the ever increasing powers of the state. Thus the term "rights" has two major historical origins and two different connotations.

Current usages of rights language reflect elements of this history. Some think of rights as privileges, as social goods that go beyond routine moral obligations. Others think of rights as a sort of social immunity, a protection from powers of the state. Rights are also seen as powers, capacities to act in society. Entitlements are another way of thinking of rights. These are social responses which are seen as deserved, as derivative from being a member of a society. Finally, rights are seen as claims, a moral demand made upon someone or on society.

Also there are different ways to think of rights. One way is to understand them as *moral*. Moral rights are based on an ethical argument and exist prior to and independent of the guarantees of any institution. Frequently these moral rights are rooted in the nature of the person and his or her dignity and are, therefore, understood to be universal and inalienable. A second type of right is *legal*—those rights spelled out by the laws, constitutions or political institutions of a particular country or political unit. Legal rights are only those rights granted to citizens by the government. They are specific to particular cultures and are subject to social qualifications. A *positive* right is a claim to a positive action on the part of another person. A positive right entails a duty on the part of someone else to do something. For example, the right of informed consent confers an obligation on the part of a health care professional to tell me relevent information about my diagnosis and treatment options. A *negative* right establishes an obligation for someone to refrain from action. Negative rights establish obligations of noninterference. The legal right to abortion, for example, does not secure an obligation for someone to perform an abortion, but only that a woman not be interfered with in seeking an abortion.

One of the most difficult problems in rights theory is establishing who is the subject of a right and on what basis. Animal rights activists argue, for example, that to have rights one need only be capable of feeling pain or be sentient. Others would suggest that consciousness is enough to secure rights. Still others argue that only self-consciousness can secure rights. Another suggestion is that one be able to use a language. This of course presents interesting issues with respect to the chimps who have been taught sign language as well as with other animals who appear to have some form of communication. Finally, the argument is made that only persons are bearers of rights. Persons are generally understood to be moral agents with an enduring concept of self and capable of autonomous actions.

The question of rights is quite complex on the level of definition and determining the subject of rights. When rights are interjected into the social order and made the basis of entitlements, then the picture becomes much more complex and difficult. We will encounter this difficulty in almost every topic we discuss in this introductory book.

Notes

1. Tom L. Beauchamp and James F. Childress, *Principles of Biomedical Ethics*. Oxford University Press, 1977, p. 56.

2. *Ibid.*, pp. 97ff.

3. For a thorough discussion of the principle of double effect, see the article "The Hermeneutical Function of the Principle of the Double Effect" by Peter Knauer, S.J. in *Readings in Moral Theology No. 1,* Charles Curran and Richard McCormick, editors. Paulist Press, 1979.

4. Richard McCormick, S.J., *Ambiguity and Moral Choice*. Department of Theology, Marquette University, p. 93.

5. Beauchamp and Childress, *op. cit.*, pp. 135ff.

6. *Ibid.*, p. 140.

7. *Ibid.*, pp 169ff.

8. *Ibid.*, pp. 66ff.

9. James Childress, *Who Shall Decide? Paternalism in Health Care*. Oxford University Press, 1982.

10. James F. Childress, *Priorities in Biomedical Ethics*. The Westminster Press, 1981, p. 27.

Discussion Questions

1. What major ethical theory do you primarily use in decision-making?

2. Do you think a health care professional has a moral obligation to care for someone with AIDS?

3. Why is the concept of informed consent so important? What functions does it perform for both patient and health care professional?

4. What method of allocation of resources seems most just to you?

5. Do you think people should have the right to refuse treatment?

6. Can you justify treating someone against his or her will?

Bibliography

Gerison Appel, *A Philosophy of Mizvot: The Religious-Ethical Concepts of Judaism. Their Roots in Biblical Tradition and the Oral Tradition.* KTAV Publishing House, 1975.

Benedict Ashley, O.P. and Kevin O'Rourke, O.P., *Health Care Ethics.* The Catholic Hospital Association, 1982.

Michael Bayles, editor, *Contemporary Utilitarianism.* Doubleday, 1968.

Charles Curran, *Themes in Fundamental Moral Theology.* University of Notre Dame Press, 1977.

———, *Issues in Sexual and Medical Ethics.* University of Notre Dame Press, 1978.

Ronald Dworkin, *Taking Rights Seriously.* Harvard University Press, 1977.

Richard Gula, *What Are They Saying About Moral Norms?* Paulist Press, 1981.

James Gustafson, *Protestant and Roman Catholic Ethics.* University of Chicago Press, 1978.

———, *Ethics from a Theocentric Perspective,* Vols. I and II. University of Chicago Press, 1981.

Stanley Hauerwas, *A Community of Character.* University of Notre Dame Press, 1981.

Alasdair MacIntyre, *After Virtue.* University of Notre Dame Press, 1981.

Daniel Maguire, *The Moral Choice.* Doubleday, 1978.

Paul Taylor, *Principles of Ethics: An Introduction.* Dickenson Publishing Co., 1975.

J. Philip Wogaman, *A Christian Method of Moral Judgment.* The Westminster Press, 1976.

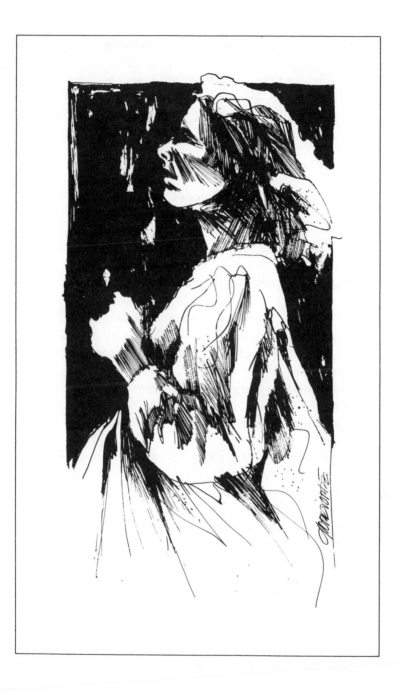

Chapter Four

ABORTION

Introduction

When *Roe v. Wade* was decided in 1973, few foresaw the impact it would have. Abortions have averaged about 1.5 million per year in the United States for the past several years. However, 1985 saw a slight decrease in the number of abortions performed. Also few suspected that the group in the United States utilizing abortion would be the teenage population, at a rate almost double that of all other Western industrial nations. The moral debate over abortion has proved to be one of the most divisive in our country's history.

The case that focuses most sharply the moral problems is the use of abortion as a back-up for contraceptive failure. When Evelyn told her husband John that she was pregnant, they faced the most serious crisis of their twelve-year marriage. Through careful planning, they had limited their family to two children, aged ten and eight. John was a bank teller and Evelyn taught high school. To enable her to pursue her career, they had used contraceptives and shared in the household responsibilities. John was shocked when Evelyn wanted an abortion.

From a legal point of view, the case is reasonably clear. No one can stop Evelyn from obtaining an abortion if she can pay for it. Morally, the issue is complex. John argued that since he would share in raising the child, he should share in the decision.

Since he was co-responsible for the conception, John said he was co-responsible for the new life. Evelyn was concerned about the impact of the birth on the welfare of the present family and her ability to continue with her career, in addition to the fact that they really chose to have no more children.

Decisions such as these have been facing literally millions of people in the last decade. And while many of the moral issues remain the same, they are no less difficult to resolve.

Legal Dimensions

Abortion legislation has covered a lot of ground since the laws of the 1800s when the test for pregnancy was quickening and abortions were prohibited only after quickening. The abortion laws that came in the mid-1800s served two functions: to establish greater control over the growing field of medicine and to control the kind of preparations used to procure abortions. In effect, some of these laws were poison control laws. In the late 1800s and early 1900s, there was a major shift in who was obtaining abortions. Typically, the immigrants had the highest use of abortion. But as their lot improved, many more gave birth. On the other hand, the women of the new native Americans were turning to abortion as a contraceptive and the population of this group began to decrease. Many of the abortion laws passed during this time were a consequence of a nativist backlash which feared that the immigrants would outnumber the new native Americans. Finally, the restrictive abortion legislation of the early and mid-twentieth century reflected a broad coalition of physicians, clergy, and the population that abortion should be controlled except for clearly defined and regulated medical circumstances, typically related to the health of the mother.[1]

Roe v. Wade,[2] decided on January 22, 1973, dramatically changed all that. This case struck down a Texas statute that made it a crime to procure or attempt an abortion except on medical advice for the purpose of saving the mother's life. This decision struck down all similar legislation in all other states. Thus was abortion decriminalized on the grounds that the right of privacy was broad enough to include a woman's decision to terminate her pregnancy. The decision also included the statement that the fetus was not a person in the sense intended by the constitution.

The second major case was *Planned Parenthood of Central Missouri v. Danforth*,[3] issued on July 1, 1976. This ruling declared unconstitutional two sections of Missouri abortion law. First, no longer could the state require the consent of the spouse for a first trimester abortion. Since the state does not have this power, neither does anyone else. Second, parents or guardians of women under eighteen cannot prohibit them from obtaining an abortion. Three reasons were given for this. First, as above, the state cannot grant to others what it itself does not have. Second, minors too have constitutional rights. Third, the state should not give parents the power to overrule a decision made by the young woman and her physician, for, in the judgment of the court, this would neither strengthen family bonds nor enhance parental authority.

The third major decision was *Beal v. Doe*,[4] issued on June 20, 1977. This decision resolved a practical point, but set off other debates. In this decision, the court held that states participating in the Medicaid program were not required to fund nontherapeutic abortions. Title 19 of the Social Security Act gives participating states broad discretionary powers in determining the extent of the medical assistance they need to provide to Medicaid recipients. The only requirement is that the standards be reasonable and consistent with the goals of Title 19. It was argued that nontherapeutic abortions were not necessary medical services and, therefore, that a refusal to fund them is not inconsistent with the aims of Title 19.

A fourth major case, *Bellotti v. Baird*,[5] decided in 1979, dealt with minors and abortion. The decision argued that every minor ought to have the opportunity to go to court without the prior consent of her parent. If the court determined that the minor was mature, it could authorize her to act without her parents' permission. If immature, she may show why the abortion is in her best interest and the court can then authorize the abortion without prior permission of the parents. Also the court may deny an abortion to a minor in the absence of parental consultation if the court judges that to be in her best interests. The basis for these rulings is that the constitutional right to have an abortion may not be unduly burdened by imposing conditions on it which hinder access to the court.

These cases have set the tone of the court decisions for the last decade. We have a different court, and new cases are being presented to it. How the justices decide these cases will have yet another significant impact on the abortion debate.

Who Is a Person?

A major part of the abortion debate has been the questions: Who is a person? By what criteria can we know this? The answer to these questions obviously has a significant impact on the evaluation of the fetus. Daniel Callahan, in his classic study of abortion, identified three basic orientations to personhood: the genetic school, the developmental school, and the school of social consequences.[6]

The genetic school defines a human person as any being that has a human genetic code. This orientation would argue that personhood comes at the beginning of life. Further growth and development are simply spelling out the implications of the genetic code for this particular individual.

The developmental school holds that while the establishment of the genetic code establishes the basis for further development, some degree of development and interaction with the environment is necessary for a being to be considered as a full human person. This orientation suggests that one's genetic potential is not fully actualized until there has been interaction with the environment. This understanding of person includes more than the biological dimension.

The third orientation is the school of social consequences which dramatically shifts the focus of the question. This orientation departs from the biological and developmental elements and focuses on what society sees as valuable for personal existence. This school first determines what kind of persons are wanted by society and then sets the definition in accordance with that. The desires of society, expressed in public policy, take precedence over the biological or developmental aspects.

Difficulties in answering the question "Who is a person?" have led to other directions. Some say that simply the capacity to experience pain or have some feelings confers rights that must be respected. Others argue that consciousness confers the entitlement of respect. Still others would require self-consciousness for such rights. Each of these orientations seeks to limit what can be done to an entity, even though that entity may not come from the formal category of person. As such these orientations broaden the criteria of rights bearers and complicate further the abortion debate.

Yet another level of complexity comes from the growing accessibility of the fetus. Such accessibility through various monitoring devices such as amniocentesis and fetoscoposy, fetal surgery, and the improvements of newborn intensive care units have allowed the fetus to be experienced as a patient. While some would argue that this is nothing new, our increased capacity to see and aid the fetus directly is a stronger basis for ascribing the status of patient than belief or ideology.

The issue is: If the fetus is a patient, is the fetus also a person? If this patient is not a person, then why treat—other than for the crassest of research motivations? If the fetus is experienced as being a person because of the status of being a patient, then what implications does that have for abortion? Major dilemmas about the personhood of the fetus are yet to be faced.

The Sanctity of Life

Another major element in the abortion debate is the concept of the sanctity of life. This phrase is a shorthand way of referring to the value of life and its inherent preciousness. Whether the value of life is external in the sense that life is a gift from the Creator or internal in that the person is an inherent center of value, the concept is an important one in thinking through the abortion dilemma.

The concept of the sanctity of life is simple in statement but complex in its explanation. The concept begins with an affirmation of the beauty and richness of biological life itself. This reflects the orientation of the Franciscan theologian Bonaventure who affirmed that creation contained the footprints of God. That which was created mirrored its Maker and, because of that, was precious.

Additionally, when that life is expressed in personal form, it takes on a new sense of mystery and value. On the one hand, following the thought of Teilhard de Chardin, we can say that personal life is creation become conscious of itself. In the person, creation is able to be aware of itself, to experience itself, to know its source and destiny. On the other hand, the distinctively human traits of intellect and will reflect what is traditionally called the image of God within the person. That is, the capacity to understand and choose reflects qualities of the divine conferred upon us in our creation. Such is the dignity of personal life: one can determine who one is and what to do and freely commit oneself to that project.

For many, such dignity is present in the member of the human species from the moment of his or her first existence. All members of the human species begin with the potential fully to express and experience personal life. What is critical in this orientation is the capacity for such development, not the actual development itself. Such capacities are not accidental to the person, but are constitutive of the essence of that person. Thus even though such potential may not be actualized—because of genetic disease or some intra-uterine trauma—such an individual is still valued because of his or her possession of life and the essential capacities of personhood.

The possession of life and the distinctively human capacities confer upon the individual an inherent value and dignity. Additionally, many affirm the innocence of such an individual. Given their initial level of personal development, they are not yet morally responsible. Additionally, these individuals are helpless, and are dependent on others for their very existence. Such absolute innocence and dependence requires, in the judgment of many, absolute protection. Only such absolute protection can be a true expression of the appreciation of the value of life.

Another approach to the concept of the sanctity of life[7] looks at it from a more social perspective. This orientation contains these elements:

(a) *Survival of the human species:* Humans ought to value their own kind and not endanger the survival of the race.

(b) *Survival of family lineage:* Families ought to be free to determine their size.

(c) *Respect for physical or bodily life:* Individuals ought to be sure of their protection and respect by others.

(d) *Respect for self-determination:* Autonomy should be respected, especially in decisions concerning health related issues.

(e) *Respect for bodily wholeness:* Individuals ought to be secure in their sense of bodily wholeness and its integrity.

If one studies these elements of the sanctity of life carefully, one can see that accepting and practicing concern for that value does not lead to clear conclusions. For example, while abortion does not promote respect for bodily life, it does not threaten the survival of the species and it helps limit the family size. Respect for the woman's self-determination and bodily wholeness may jeopardize those values for the fetus. Thus sometimes adherence to the value and significance of the sanctity of life causes individuals to be on opposite sides of the abortion debate and to hold conflicting values. Individuals become adversaries as they each try to implement and promote reverence for the sanctity of life.

Finally, it is important to think about how one relates the issue of ending life in abortion and ending life in other situations. Many moral and/or religious ethical theories have permitted or promoted killing in some circumstances: self-defense, the defense of private property, war, capital punishment. Here the value of life—the sanctity of life—is balanced off against other important values: personal bodily integrity, the right to keep what is one's own, democracy, freedom, the security of society. The moral issue frequently is not whether we may kill, but under what circumstances killing is permitted.

Some respond to this situation by total pacifism, by prohibiting any killing or violence in any fashion in any circumstances. Others set up categories such as the just war theory that helps define a narrow range of circumstances in which killing is permitted. Others declare certain kinds of killing off limits: abortion and direct euthanasia. Each solution brings certain problems to the solution it provided to the moral problem of killing, but each also does its best to promote the sanctity of life.

Three Positions on Abortion

When all is said and done, there are three basic orientations to abortion: the conservative, the liberal, and the moderate.[8] The conservative position holds that under no circumstances may an abortion be performed. The religious and philosophical reasons for this include: the sanctity of life, the inviolability of innocent human life, and the fear of the social implications of a liberal abortion policy for other defenseless people such as the handicapped and the elderly.

The liberal position would allow abortion under many different circumstances. Many individuals see abortion as a moral decision, but assume a broad range of moral justifications. These include: the quality of life of the fetus, the physical and mental health status of the woman, her rights to bodily integrity, the welfare of the existing family, career considerations, and family planning.

The moderate position seeks a middle ground which recognizes the moral legitimacy of some abortions, but never without suffering and pain on the part of both the woman and fetus. This position sees both the fetus and woman as having rights and entitlements and recognizes that attempts to resolve such conflicts of rights will entail suffering and pain. Thus, while accepting the moral acceptability of some abortions, the moderates accept this only with a sense of great tragedy and loss.

Two World Views

Gregory Baum identifies the cause for the profound disagreements and moral conflicts presented in this chapter as rooted in radically different world views on nature and sexuality.[9] The first world view sees sexuality and reproduction as part of nature. They are defined by divine providence as having a primarily biological function which, while being pleasurable, is intrinsically related to reproduction. Since nature is defined and watched over by the Creator, interference in that order through artificial contraception or abortion is a violation of that order. Such an orientation would typically be conservative on the abortion question.

The second orientation sees God's providence expressed, not in a static understanding of the biological order, but rather as gracious action within human history which enables people to take more responsibility for themselves and their environment. Sexuality is more than biology; it is a personal act and a human reality with many dimensions. Contraception is a means of exercising responsibility, not violating a biological order. Abortion also becomes a moral possibility in this perspective.

Such differences in world view cannot explain all differences between people. However they can help reveal why people disagree so much. They begin at different points, and they may be unaware of this until they are pushed back to some basic perspective. Thus the most profound area of disagreement may not be over how to resolve a specific moral issue such as abortion, but over our assumptions about how much responsibility individuals have and whether or not the biological order can be altered. These perspectives define the context in which individuals make moral decisions and shape their understanding of moral accountability.

The Public Policy Debate

Another major problem in the abortion debate is related to the basis on which public policy is debated. The themes developed here are relevant for other policy issues, but come into particularly sharp focus on abortion.

Alasdair MacIntyre[10] argues that morality is at war with itself because each moral agent reaches conclusions by valid forms of inference but cannot agree about the correctness or appropriateness of the premise with which the argument begins. This means that we can agree on valid forms or structures of an argument, but we cannot agree on the proper or appropriate starting point.

There are two major reasons for this. First, we have not inherited the social or cultural context in which we can both understand and apply a particular philosophical theory. Our use of a philosophical theory is separate from the culture which gave birth to it and nurtured it. Second, we have inherited conflicting theories of ethics and social philosophy. Ours is a culture which has many definitions, theories and methods of ethics, few of which lead to conclusions consistent with each other. Each presents conflicting and even contrary claims with respect to what is good for humans and how humans relate to the community.

For example, the classical tradition asks the question: How might humans together realize the common good? The modern tradition asks: How might humans prevent each other from interfering with one another as each goes about his or her concerns? The first question assumes that humans can know and agree upon what is good for all. The second question assumes that what is good for me might not be good for you. If people approach each other with such conflicting assumptions about human nature and the relation of humans in society, how can major policy issues be addressed in a coherent fashion? Knowledge of such disparate points of view, while not making the debate any easier, at least helps us realize why all do not emerge at the same place.

These are some of the thematic issues that Evelyn and John must face in discussing their pregnancy. Each will have to be faced thoroughly and honestly. Each will have to be evaluated in the light of all the other perspectives we have discussed. No matter what the decision, pain, tragedy and a sense of loss will occur. Such is the nature of the abortion debate.

Notes

1. For a thorough discussion of the development of abortion legislation in America, see James C. Mohr, *Abortion in America: The Origins and the Evolution of National Policy.* Oxford University Press, 1978.

2. 410 U.S. 113.

3. 96 S. Ct. 2831.

4. 97 S. Ct. 2366.

5. 99 S. Ct. 3035.

6. Daniel Callahan, *Abortion: Law, Choice and Morality.* Macmillan, 1970, pp. 378ff.

7. *Ibid.,* pp. 307ff.

8. James Nelson, *Human Medicine.* Augsburg Publishing House, 1973, pp. 31ff.

9. Gregory Baum, "Abortion: An Ecumenical Dilemma," *Commonweal* 30 (November 1973) 231–235.

10. Alaisdair MacIntyre, "How To Identify Ethical Principles," *The Belmont Report,* Appendix, Vol. 1. DHEW Publication No. (OSO 78-0013, 10-1-41).

Topics for Discussion

1. Is the sanctity of life compatible with the taking of life?
2. Many people argue that one should be consistent in one's

position on killing. That is, if one is against abortion, then one should be against war or capital punishment. Do you agree? How would you make exceptions.?

3. What are the strengths and weaknesses of each of the major definitions of a person indicated in the chapter?

4. Does the argument of the moderate position on abortion work? How do you justify your response to this?

5. How would you advise Evelyn and John? What are your reasons for this advice?

Bibliography

W. B. Bondeson *et al.*, editors, *Abortion and the Status of the Fetus*. D. Reidel Publishing Co., 1983.

Daniel Callahan, *Abortion: Law, Choice and Morality*. Macmillan, 1970.

Sidney and Daniel Callahan, *Abortion: Understanding Differences*. Plenum, 1984.

John Connery, S.J., *Abortion: The Development of the Roman Catholic Perspective*. Loyola University Press, 1977.

Germaine Griesez, *Abortion: The Myths, the Realities and the Arguments*. World Publishing Company, 1970.

Beverly Harrison, *Our Right To Choose: Toward a New Ethic of Abortion*. Beacon Press, 1983.

Kristen Lucker, *Abortion and the Politics of Motherhood*. University of California Press, 1984.

James Mohr, *Abortion in America: The Origins and Evolution of National Policy*. Oxford University Press, 1974.

John T. Noonan, Jr., *The Morality of Abortion: Legal and Historical Perspectives*. Harvard University Press, 1970.

Malcolm Potts *et al.*, *Abortion*. Cambridge University Press, 1977.

Margery W. Shaw *et al.*, editors, *Defining Human Life: Medical, Legal, and Ethical Implications*. AUPHA Press, 1983.

David Thomasma, *An Apology for the Value of Human Life*. St. Louis Catholic Health Association, 1983.

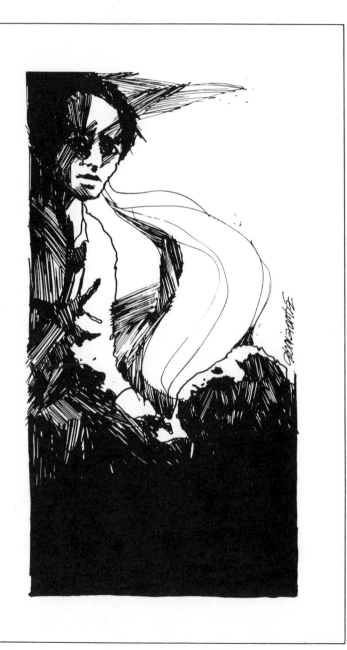

Chapter Five

THE DEFINITION OF DEATH

General Introduction

One of the most critical moments in the life of an individual is the end of that life. But ironically much confusion has surrounded that moment. On the one hand, Phillipe Aries has described the ritual of death in which the one dying took formal leave of his or her loved one and the community. But on the other hand, the moment of death frequently was uncertain. There is a literature reflecting the fear of being buried alive. Various technical interventions such as breathing tubes or bells were attached to coffins so that someone mistakenly buried alive could signal others. The morgue originally was a place to observe bodies to ensure that the individual was in fact dead.

Many of these problems were overcome or softened by certain realities, however. First, few medicines were available to help people overcome illnesses. Second, no technical interventions were present to prolong life. Third, since the life span was short—forty years would have been considered a ripe old age even a hundred years ago—people were more accepting of death as a fact of life. Thus when people became ill, they died, and they died within a community context that supported their dying.

Perhaps the major difference between an older age and ours is found in a petition from the Litany of Saints: "From a sudden and unprovided death, deliver us, O Lord." To die without a formal leave taking, without reconciliation, without putting one's affairs in order, without an acknowledgement of the end was a personal and communal tragedy for previous generations. Today, however, most would want a sudden and rapid death, preferably a death which would catch one unaware. While people surely would want to have their affairs in order, most seem to want more a rapid end because of a fear of a lingering, out of control death.

The shift in orientation has several reasons. First, our life span has increased dramatically in the last several generations. Individuals can now expect to live until their mid-70s or even longer. Second, modern medicine has succeeded in eliminating many of the diseases that would routinely destroy whole populations. Third, and perhaps most critically, our generation has the technical capacity to intervene and prolong the dying process with various life support systems.

The use of respirators and other life support systems has raised significant problems with respect to defining death. These technical interventions mask or hide the traditional criteria in use for the past several generations: spontaneous breathing and heartbeat. That is, if one uses the absence of breathing and heartbeat as the sign of death, how do these criteria apply when one is on a respirator? When a respirator is breathing for an individual, in what sense, if any, is that person alive? In what sense, if any, can that person be considered dead? Thus the need for an examination of the definition of death is pressed upon us.

Four Approaches to a Definition

The framework developed by Robert Veatch for examining various definitions of death is still useful.[1] The framework helps us identify significant issues, makes us aware of the consequences of a particular definition, and helps us be precise in evaluating various criteria for validating the definition.

Heart and lung. Veatch's first definition reflects the traditional understanding of life and death. Since breath and blood are the stuff of life, their absence marks the presence of death. When the vital signs are absent, death has occurred. But it is this traditional definition that has been clouded by the use of the respirator. Who is responsible for the vital signs: the person or the respirator?

Separation of body and soul. The second definition emerges from a philosophical and religious perspective. This definition, based on the philosophy of Aristotle, understands the person as a unity of body and soul or matter and form. The soul or form animates the body or matter, creating the unique entity that we know as the person. Death occurs when these two elements are separated. Death is the dissolution of the union of body and soul. The main problem with this definition is how to test whether the union is dissolved. Such a problem is implicitly recognized in the Roman Catholic pastoral practice which allows clergy to administer conditionally the last rites up to several hours after an "official" pronouncement of death, especially if the death was the result of an accident.

Veatch's third and fourth definitions are responses to the dilemmas of defining death posed by technical interventions into the dying process. Thus, as mentioned, a respirator can mask the inability to spontaneously breathe. Also a person in an irreversible coma or a chronically persistent vegetative stage can have physical life extended by use of various life support systems. The intensive care unit is a symbol of the tremendous success of modern medicine because many lives which would have been lost are routinely saved. But it is also a symbol of the dilemmas of modern medicine in that often the best that technology can do is to either maintain the status quo or prolong the dying that will inevitably occur. Thus the need for new definitions and criteria arise.

Brain dead. Definition three is derived from the standards for irreversible coma drawn up by an ad hoc committee at the

Harvard Medical School in 1969.[2] These criteria—unreceptivity and unresponsiveness, no spontaneous movements or breathing, no reflexes, with the confirmation of this situation by an electroencephalogram—seek to give a means of confirming a total and irreversible lack of activity in the brain. In this orientation, the brain is the locus of death because it is the organ which integrates all other organ systems and is the basis for one's social presence in the world. The death of the brain or its irreversible loss of a capacity to function removes the biological pre-condition for the person's existence. The death of the whole brain (the brain stem, the cortex, and the neocortex) is equated with the death of the person because without this organ the person has no means of being biologically and therefore also socially integrated.

Neocortical dead. One problem yet remains. Only the brain stem of a person, typically someone in an irreversible coma, may be operative. Since the brain stem is responsible for our involuntary nervous system, this individual may be spontaneously breathing and the heart beating on its own. According to definition three, this individual is not dead. Definition four addresses this situation by looking only to the neocortex as the locus for a definition of death. The neocortex is selected because the neocortex appears to be the biological pre-condition for consciousness and self-awareness, distinctive personal characteristics. Since the biological basis for self-awareness is gone, the person is no longer an integrated social whole. The person is dead even though, paradoxically, physical life still goes on. By using this definition we are confronted with a cadaver which is still breathing. The disposition of such a cadaver presents tremendous religious, philosophical, and psychological problems.

These attempts to define and redefine death raise critical problems and catch us up in profound debates with extremely significant consequences. However, as long as dying continues to occur in a technological context, these definitions will continue to be debated.

The Limits of Responsibility

The redefining of death evokes awesome responsibilities. Some have suggested that such attempts to redefine death are well beyond the responsibilities humans have. Others argue that we have no choice since not to decide is also to decide. Since there are limits to medicine, we must make a virtue of necessity and establish reasonable criteria. However in doing this we will be well advised to keep in mind the sage advice of Paul Ramsey that while there may be limits to curing, there are never limits to caring.[3]

One common objection to redefining death is that it is "playing God," appropriating to humans what is the responsibility of God alone. This objection is based on the traditional understanding of God as the Author of life and death. Hence, death is God's responsibility and interferences with it are overstepping the limits of human responsibility. Such a view, first, confuses defining death with the authority to take life. The purpose of defining death is to determine when it has occurred, not to take a person's life. Second, this view uncritically, or perhaps naively, assumes that God is directly and immediately involved in each and every physical or biological event in the universe. While wanting to avoid the position that God created the world and then left it to its own devices, we must also reject the contrary position which assumes that God directs each and every act occurring in the world. The former view overstates human responsibility; the latter devalues it.

A second problem comes from the very practical issue of what to do with people in irreversible comas or chronic vegetative states. On the one hand, individuals in such conditions can be maintained almost indefinitely. On the other hand, if we do maintain such individuals, our intensive care units become overburdened. Individuals who need an ICU as a transitional phase of their recovery may be at risk of not being admitted because of the unit's being overcrowded. Thus considerations of space and economics force the question of the status of these individuals upon us. Also our own ethical concern for respect for persons causes us to examine their situation. A person can be just as much violated by overtreatment as undertreatment. We have a moral obligation to treat a cadaver with respect, but not to continue to provide it with expensive medical therapies. Thus a re-examination of the definition of death can provide us with an orientation to some of these problems.

Third, we need to consider the issue of suffering. Although suffering is an evil and is one of the major problems of human existence, we have nonetheless attempted to find meaning in it, again making a virtue of necessity. Some see suffering as contributing to the development of character, as strengthening one's personality. The discipline learned from suffering allows one to make one's way through the world and succeed. Others experience suffering in a religious context and see it as a means of transforming the self and the community. Such an experience of redemptive suffering can be an occasion for personal growth and the strengthening of the community. All of us know the inspiration derived from experiencing such an understanding of suffering.

Yet, when a person is comatose, when an individual cannot personalize the suffering or in some way appropriate the suffering to oneself, may not such suffering simply be impersonal, unredemptive, meaningless? Thus, although one may wish to and, in fact, may succeed in making suffering a religious experience or an occasion for personal growth, may there not come a time or situation in which such efforts cease? The patient is in a coma and cannot respond to the situation. The family cannot interact with the patient. Little or no sense can be made of the situation; growth and development can no longer occur. Such destructive suffering may lead to the despair of all.

New Directions

Personal and technical considerations which have given rise to attempts to redefine death continue to be with us. Such efforts seek to come to terms with the limits of medicine in seeking to cure an individual. They seek to respect the rights of individuals and to maintain their dignity by prohibiting over-treatment or inappropriate treatment. Thus the redefinition of death is an attempt to resolve the limbo-like situations of the irreversibly comatose patient in an honest and forthright manner.

The continued press of events, ongoing debates on the appropriateness of various definitions of death, and the continuing problems presented by life support systems led to formal consideration of death by a presidential commission: The President's Commission for the Study of Ethical Problems in Medicine and Biomedical and Behavioral Research. This commission, recognizing that many states had legislated differing definitions of death, proposed a uniform standard.

The commission reached its conclusion about the definition of death and its implementation based on several considerations.

1. Recent developments mandate such considerations.
2. Thus a restatement ought to be a matter of statutory law.
3. Such laws ought to be, at present, enacted on the state level.
4. Such laws ought to be uniform.
5. The definition ought to address physiological standards rather than medical tests and criteria that can be outdated by new knowledge and technical developments.
6. Death is a unitary phenomenon and can be determined by either traditional heart-lung criteria or brain criteria. This helps avoid perceptions of different degrees of death.
7. Definitions of death ought be kept separate from provisions concerning organ donation and decisions to withhold or withdraw life support systems.[4]

Given these considerations as well as the conclusions of various other studies, the commission recommended the following as a uniform definition of death: "An individual who has sustained either (1) irreversible cessation of circulatory and respiratory function, or (2) irreversible cessation of all function of the entire brain, including the brain stem, is dead. A determination of death must be made in accordance with accepted medical standards."[5]

The strength of this proposed definition is that it recognizes—to put it directly—that when you are dead, you are dead, regardless of which definition is used. Thus brain death has the same validity as traditional cardio-pulmonary death. Also the definition does not lock anyone into the technology or knowledge of a particular time. The criteria for determining death are the responsibility of the medical profession and will change as knowledge and technology change.

This recommendation will set the tone for future discussions. The commission has provided a framework for analysis, a location for determining criteria, and a validation of the concept that death is one, regardless of where one locates it. While not resolving all of the difficult and frequently tragic circumstances that surround death and its defining, the commission orients us to an understanding that can help us resolve many of our difficulties.

Notes

1. Robert M. Veatch, *Death, Dying and the Biological Revolution.* Yale University Press, 1976, pp. 21ff.

2. Ad Hoc Committee of the Harvard Medical School, "A Definition of Irreversible Coma," *Journal of the American Medical Association* 205 (August 1968) 337–40.

3. Paul Ramsey, *The Patient as Person.* Yale University Press, 1970.

4. President's Commission for the Study of Ethical Problems in Medicine and Biomedical and Behavioral Research, *Defining Death: Medical, Legal and Ethical Issues in the Determination of Death.* U.S. Government Printing Office, 1981.

5. *Ibid.,* pp. 1–2.

Discussion Questions

1. Why has defining death become so difficult?
2. What kinds of technical resources complicate defining death? How do they do this?
3. What are some of the social implications of redefining death?
4. Who should be responsible for redefining death?
5. Do you think the President's Commission should have adopted a neo-cortical definition of death?

Bibliography

Ad Hoc Committee, Harvard University Medical School, "A Definition of Irreversible Coma," *Journal of the American Medical Association* 205 (1968) 337–340.

Tom Beauchamp and Seymour Perlin, eds., *Ethical Issues in Death and Dying.* Prentice-Hall, 1978.

James L. Bernat *et al.,* "Defining Death in Theory and Practice," *The Hastings Center Report* 12 (February 1982) 5–9.

Paul A. Byrne *et al.,* "Brain Death: An Opposing Viewpoint," *Journal of the American Medical Association* 242 (1979) 1985.

Alexander M. Capron and Leon R. Kass, "A Statutory Definition of the Standards for Determining Human Death: An Appraisal and a Proposal," *University of Pennsylvania Law Review* 121 (1972) 87ff.

Peter McL. Black, "Brain Death," *The New England Journal of Medicine* 299 (1978) 338 and 393.

President's Commission for the Study of Ethical Problems in Medicine and Biomedical and Behavioral Research, *Defining Death: Medical, Legal and Ethical Issues in the Determination of Death.* U.S. Government Printing Office, 1981.

Task Force of the Hastings Center, "Refinements in the Criteria for the Determination of Death," *Journal of the American Academy of Medicine* 221 (July 9, 1972) 48–53.

Frank Veith *et al.*, "Brain Death: I: A Status Report of Medical and Ethical Considerations." "II: A Status Report of Legal Considerations." *Journal of the American Medical Association* 238 (October 10 and 17, 1977) 1651–1655, 1744–1748.

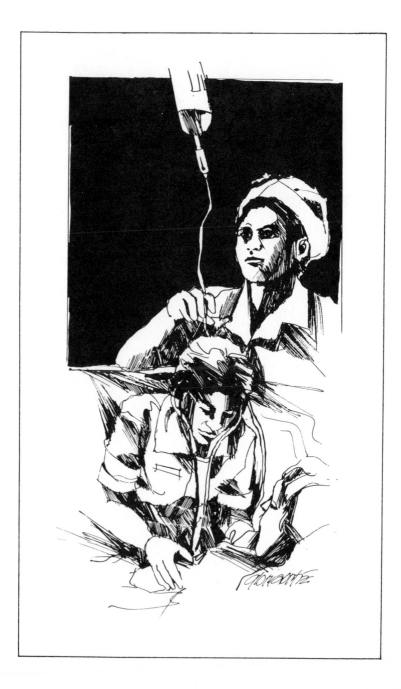

Chapter Six

EUTHANASIA

Introduction

Two major factors control our perception of dying. First, the diseases or problems associated with growing older are proving very difficult to cure. Various debilitations associated with senility, different forms of cancer, and Alzheimer's disease ultimately bring about death, but frequently only after a long-drawn-out process of suffering. Second, while individuals are in this debilitated state, their lives—or dying—can be prolonged by technical interventions. Such interventions cannot cure—nor were they designed to. However, once an individual is on a life support system, many individuals are reluctant to remove that individual from it.

These problems, perceptions and experiences of being trapped on machines as well as genuine concern for those whose dying is being prolonged have caused euthanasia to be considered anew. Some see euthanasia as an end to intolerable suffering or a hopeless situation. Others see it as a way of easing a transition that is already occurring. Still others see it as anticipating the inevitable. Euthanasia is also seen as a right or an entitlement, a person's last expression of human dignity. Homicide is still another way of understanding euthanasia. It is an unjustified usurpation of power to oneself, an overstepping of the bounds of the stewardship of one's body.

Public events have given publicity to euthanasia also. In 1984, Governor Lamm of Colorado suggested that older citizens may have a duty to die so that they will not deplete scarce resources for others. Elizabeth Bouvia, a twenty-six year old cerebral palsy victim, asked to be allowed to starve herself to death. And in 1985, Roswell Gilbert became the first individual convicted of homicide for an act of direct euthanasia. Mrs. Gilbert suffered from Alzheimer's disease and osteoporosis that left her disoriented and in considerable pain. After she told her husband that she wanted to die, he shot her. Finally, Karen Ann Quinlan's death on June 11, 1985, ten years after being disconnected from a respirator, focused attention again on the ethical dilemmas associated with withdrawing life support systems.

A distinction between voluntary and involuntary euthanasia must be made before the consideration of the ethics of euthanasia. Voluntary euthanasia is euthanasia performed either by or at the request of the recipient of the act. Involuntary euthanasia is performed without the consent of the individual.

Although voluntary euthanasia is frequently discussed in connection with the ethics of suicide, there are two reasons for keeping the discussion separate. First, suicide is typically an interruption in the life process and occurs in a non-medical context. Second, euthanasia is an anticipation of imminent or certain death from a disease.

Involuntary euthanasia is complicated by the fact that the patient is incompetent. Thus the patient has no say in the matter. And even though the patient may have indicated his or her wishes before lapsing into unconsciousness, euthanasia still requires another individual actively to intervene to end another's life.

Another distinction—direct and indirect—is of importance in discussing euthanasia and will serve as the basis for the next sections of this chapter.

Direct or Active Euthanasia

In direct or active euthanasia, whether voluntary or involuntary, death is the goal of one's actions. The intervention—an overdose of sleeping pills, an injection of poison—is intended to end the life of the patient. This direct relation between intent and motive is the basic reason why many consider direct euthanasia another form of homicide.

The major reason why people oppose direct euthanasia is that since God is the Creator and alone has full dominion over life and death, such a taking of life is an overstepping of human responsibility. Humans are stewards of their lives and, as such, have limited control over what they may do.

This opposition to euthanasia is closely related to the rejection of abortion based on the sanctity of life arguments we discussed before. Because life is inherently precious and valuable, no one under any circumstances may end it.

Third, many oppose direct or active euthanasia because of fear of getting on to the slippery slope. If one allows killing the dying or the irreversibly comatose—for whatever good motive—what is to stop us from expanding the categories and killing newborns, the mentally ill, the retarded, the unproductive, the socially undesirable? Once the barriers to direct killing are expanded, then no one is safe.

Fourth, if active or direct euthanasia becomes acceptable, this may have a detrimental effect on the relation between patients and physicians and on the perceptions of health care facilities. If seriously ill persons know that physicians or hospitals could administer direct euthanasia, individuals might be reluctant to be treated or even to enter such facilities.

On the other hand, several arguments are put forward supporting active euthanasia. First, if a person is dying and nothing can be done, why should a person not be able to choose death now rather than later. The point here is that the person is dying and the act of euthanasia anticipates what will inevitably happen.

Second, if the only means of controlling patients' pain is to keep them unconscious, or if patients are in a irreversible coma, then why not end their misery? These are individuals for whom nothing can be done except to maintain the status quo. Intervening directly to end their lives will end their misery.

Third, such situations of helplessness and hopelessness take a serious toll on the family of patients. The inability of a family to do anything for their relative may cause pain and suffering almost as great as that experienced by the patient. Also the dramatically increasing costs of medical care may totally deplete the resources of a family within days or weeks. Thus direct euthanasia is justified because of the helpless condition of the patient and the greater good of the other family members.

Direct or active euthanasia—because it is an active ending of a person's life—raises serious moral difficulties. But the context of these difficulties—the hopelessness of a patient's condition—is also an important moral consideration. Thus the ethical debate on direct euthanasia is between motive—mercy—and rule—do not murder.

Indirect or Passive Euthanasia

Indirect or passive euthanasia attempts to resolve many of the problems of the moral treatment of the hopelessly ill or dying by withdrawing therapies so that the natural chain of events can occur. In this orientation, one omits acts or removes therapies so that one will not impede what is inevitable—the patient's death. In passive or indirect euthanasia, the patient's death is forseen, but not aimed at or intended. Assumedly, removing a respirator will contribute to an individual's death, and the health care team and family know this. However the important moral difference is that the cause of death is the disease process at work in the patient, not the acts of the family or health care team.

The moral consideration of passive or indirect euthanasia

has a long and complex history. And the continued use of technological interventions in medicine has raised other issues. A review of several of these dilemmas will help us sort out some of the problems.

Ordinary and extraordinary means of treatment

These terms refer to a way of categorizing treatments or therapies. Ordinary therapies typically referred to medicines, treatments, or operations which offered a reasonable amount of benefit to a patient and could be obtained without excessive pain, expense, or other inconvenience. Extraordinary therapies were those which, while offering little benefit, were very costly, very painful and exceptionally inconvenient.[1] The standard moral rule was that one was obligated to use only those treatments which were ordinary; otherwise too high an ethical standard would be imposed on individuals.

Technical interventions in medicine have complicated this traditional distinction particularly with respect to its use in classifying treatment modalities. First, the rapid incorporation of a technology into standard or ordinary medical practice makes it difficult to classify a technology as extraordinary. Respirators and dialysis machines are expensive, but they are a standard part of medical practice. Second, judgments of whether a treatment is ordinary or not have more to do with value judgments about the technology than the technology in itself. Thus for a Jehovah's Witness, a blood transfusion is extraordinary while for all others it is routine. For most, a highly experimental therapy for cancer may be extraordinary because of its side-effects, but for those who want to increase their life span, it may be ordinary.

These difficulties have led many to propose dropping the terms ordinary and extraordinary as a means of *classifying* treatments which would then determine their moral appropriateness. Rather, the terms are useful as a way of assessing the consequences of a treatment. Thus they are seen as the *conclusion* of an argument about the type of therapy proposed or an *evaluation* of the consequences of a treatment. Contemporary usage favors retaining the evaluative dimension of the original definitions, but eliminating their classificatory elements.

Actions and omissions that lead to death

This distinction goes to the heart of the moral justification of passive euthanasia. As the recent Presidential Commission states it: "The distinction between a fatal act and a fatal omission depends both upon the difference between a person physically acting and refraining from acting and upon what might be called the background course of events."[2] At issue is the moral validity of an act of omission that one knows will set a context leading to an individual's death. Also critical is the agent's intention: the omission of a useless or burdensome treatment—not the intention directly to cause death.

This Commission also identified four typical differences between fatal acts and omissions that are helpful in evaluating the morality of omitting treatment.[3]

1. The motives of an agent who acts to cause death are usually worse (for example, self-interest or malice) than those of someone who omits to act and lets another die.

2. A person who is barred from acting to cause another's death is usually thereby placed at no personal risk of harm, whereas, especially outside the medical context, if a person were forced to intercede to save another's life (instead of standing by and omitting to act), he or she could often be put at a substantial risk.

3. The nature and duration of future life denied to a person whose life is ended by another's act is usually much greater than that denied to a dying person whose death comes slightly more quickly due to an omission of treatment.

4. A person, especially a patient, may still have some possibility of surviving if one omits to act, while survival is more often foreclosed by actions that lead to death.

These perspectives help us consider the consequences of our acts, evaluate the burdens imposed by a continuing of the status quo, and judge the relation between our proposals and the patient's values and goals.

This distinction also raises the issues of the causality of the death. When we act to cause death—by injecting a poison into the patient—the causal agent is the poison and we are the ones who administered it. We are the cause of death because had we not done what we did, the patient would not have then died. On the other hand, if we omit to do something—do not provide cardiac resuscitation—then we assume that the cause of death is the underlying disease. This is the case even though the patient would not have died had we provided resuscitation.

Such considerations about causality are comforting although they might not give an account of the moral appropriateness of the omission. However, as the President's Commission notes: "Consequently, these distinctions, while often conceptually unclear and of dubious moral importance in themselves, are useful in facilitating acceptance of sound decisions that would otherwise meet unwarranted resistance. They help people involved to understand, in ways acceptable to them, their proper roles in implementing decisions to forego life-sustaining treatment."[4]

Withholding and withdrawing treatment

This distinction is related to the action/omission distinction because frequently people feel that withdrawing an already initiated therapy is acting, while not starting a therapy is analogous to an act of omission. Generally speaking, the moral arguments for either are typically identical. That is, the reasons for not initiating a respirator frequently are the same as the arguments for withdrawing it. And these arguments have to do with the patient's values, expected benefits of the action, or the burdens of the treatment. And again the issue of intentionality enters here. If the intention is to withhold or withdraw a useless or burdensome treatment, the act is typically justified, whereas if the intention is to end the patient's life, the act is typically unjustified.

The major differences have to do with the expectations

aroused in the patient, family and medical team from the initia-
tion of a therapy, the momentum that develops and intensifies
during therapy, and the all too common and universal
unwillingness to admit failure. Thus while most will frequently
agree that a therapy is doing little, if any, good for the patient,
disagreement will frequently arise about the appropriateness of
withdrawing the therapy primarily because it signifies the
inability of anybody to do anything for the patient. Thus the
moral issue once again is the evaluation of the benefits and
burdens of the therapy on the patient.

Intended and unintended but foreseeable consequences

Pain relievers such as morphine achieve their goal—but at
a cost. While relieving pain, they make breathing difficult. This
raises the question of the moral appropriateness of using increasing levels of morphine to control pain while knowing that
this will eventually cause the patient's death.

One issue that is morally important is intention. If the
intention is to kill the patient, then we have surely crossed a line
and are talking about euthanasia—or homicide. If the intention
is relief of pain, such an action is located within the context of
medical care. It is this difference in intention—not burdening
the patient with a futile or extraordinarily burdensome treatment—that marks the difference between unjustified active
euthanasia and justified passive euthanasia.

Second, one needs to acknowledge that such actions put the
patient at the risk of death, and one has to consider whether
there are less risky means available to achieve the same end. In
this regard, the Commission notes: "The degree of care and
judgment exercised by the physician should therefore be guided
not only by the broader question of whether care providers are
certain enough of the facts in this case, including the patient's
priorities and subjective experience, to risk death in order to
relieve suffering. If this can be answered affirmatively, there is
no moral or legal objection to using the kinds and amounts of
drugs necessary to relieve the patient's pain."[5]

Summary

Considerations of direct and indirect euthanasia and the other distinctions discussed in this chapter should have convinced us of one thing: the issue is complex and difficult. Many critical value issues are raised, as well as issues of professional and familial responsibility. The elements considered in this chapter provide a way into the ethical dilemmas surrounding the treatment of the terminally ill or the dying, but they do not give an easy or mechanical formula for resolving these demanding issues. As the Commission notes: "The acceptability of particular actions or omissions turns on other morally significant considerations, such as the balance of harms and benefits likely to be achieved, the duties owed by others to a dying person, the risks imposed on them in acting or refraining, and the certainty of outcome."[6]

Notes

1. Gerald Kelly, S.J., *Medico-Moral Problems*. The Catholic Hospital Association, 1958, p. 129.
2. President's Commission for the Study of Ethical Problems in Medicine and Biomedical and Behavioral Research, *Deciding To Forego Life-Sustaining Treatment*. U.S. Government Printing Office, 1983, p. 65.
3. *Ibid.*, p. 66.
4. *Ibid.*, p. 71.
5. *Ibid.*, p. 81.
6. *Ibid.*, p. 61.

Topics for Discussion

1. Do you think the distinction between euthanasia and suicide is relevant?
2. Is there a moral difference between direct and indirect euthanasia?

3. What are the ethical risks involved in letting someone die?

4. Do you agree that the arguments for withholding treatment are the same as those for withdrawing treatment?

5. Do you agree with the acceptance of the practice of giving increasing levels of pain relievers, even though they may cause the death of the patient?

6. Much controversy has surrounded the possibility of withdrawing or withholding food and water. Are food and water ordinary or extraordinary means of treatment? Are they forms of treatment? Is this analogous to withdrawing or withholding a respirator?

Bibliography

John A. Behnke and Sissela Bok, *The Dilemma of Euthanasia.* Doubleday Anchor, 1975.

Lisa S. Cahill. "A 'Natural Law' Reconsideration of Euthanasia," *Linacre Quarterly* 44 (February 1977) 47–63.

A. B. Downing, *Euthanasia and the Right To Die.* Humanities Press, 1970.

Richard M. Gula, S.S., *What Are They Saying About Euthanasia?* Paulist Press, 1986.

Dennis J. Horan and David Mall, editors, *Death, Dying and Euthanasia.* University Publications of America, 1977.

David Lester *et al.,* editors, *Suicide: A Guide to Information Sources.* Gale Research Company, 1980.

Daniel Maguire, *Death By Choice.* Doubleday, Revised Edition, 1984.

Albert S. Moracewski and J. Stuart Showalter, *Determination of Death.* Catholic Health Association, 1982.

President's Commission, *Deciding To Forego Life-Sustaining Treatment.* U.S. Government Printing Office, 1983.

James Rachels, "Active and Passive Euthanasia," *The New England Journal of Medicine* 292 (January 9, 1975) 78–80.

Ruth O. Russell, *Freedom To Die: Moral and Legal Aspects of Euthanasia*. Human Sciences Press, 1975.

David E. Stannard, editor, *Death in America*. University of Pennsylvania Press, 1975.

Robert M. Veatch, *Death, Dying and the Biological Revolution*. Yale University Press, 1976.

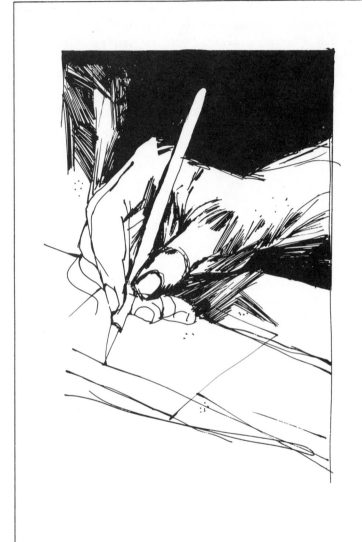

Chapter Seven

THE LIVING WILL

Introduction

Concerns about how to ensure one's wishes about the disposal of property, money, possessions, and even one's body have been fairly constant concerns of people. Historically, these and similar problems have been resolved through one's last will and testament, a legally sanctioned instrument which ensures that one's wishes will be carried out after death.

Developments in technology which ensure one's physical survival but not necessarily one's recovery have raised questions about treatment decisions which need to be made when the patient is incompetent and perhaps likely to remain so. Previous chapters have indicated several orientations and problems with respect to decision-making. This chapter will examine another solution: the living will.

In general, the concept of the living will proposes that, while competent, we indicate our wishes about how we wish to be treated in the event that we become incompetent. The living will seeks to keep responsibility for decision-making with the patient. In this way, control over specific issues—for example, whether the patient should be physically maintained, what is in the patient's best interest, and who is the decision-maker—is centered on the patient, as it is in all other situations.

The Karen Ann Quinlan case alerted us to how difficult and

draining such decision-making can be—both on the personal and social level. For while it is the case that frequently patients are unable to decide for themselves, nonetheless decisions must be made. Issues of scarcity of resources, the cost of intensive care units, the best interests of the patient, and a host of value issues are raised and make it imperative that a decision be made—and often made rather quickly. The living will affirms that the responsibility for such decision-making is the patient's and provides a means for exercising the responsibility.

The philosophy of the living will reflects three cornerstones of contemporary medical ethics. First, the doctrine of informed consent defines the patient as the decision-maker. Second, there is a common ethical and religious sanctioning of the legitimacy of refusing extraordinary, heroic, or nonbeneficial treatments. Third, all competent patients have a legal right to refuse treatment. The living will is an attempt to ensure that a patient can exercise these rights by declaring in advance, when competent, how he or she wishes to be treated in the event of incompetency. Thus the only new element in the concept of the living will is that one's advance declarations about treatment decisions be honored. Everything else is in accord with traditional medical ethics.

Some Problems

Of course what is novel about the living will is what causes the problems. For example, how do we know that the individual had not changed his or her mind about the treatment decision? Was the patient competent when the will was made? Did the patient envision his or her present circumstances when making the will? How binding on the family and/or health care team is the living will? What is its legal status?

Obviously, when people are unconscious it is impossible to ask them whether they have changed their mind or not. Family or friends may be asked to help by reporting on recent conversations, but a direct answer is impossible. On the other hand, if an individual has taken the time to make the effort to draw up or sign such a will, this should constitute acceptable evidence that the individual is serious about its contents. Thus support of the will, absent any contradictory evidence, is reasonable.

Again, questions about the person's competence when drafting the will may be difficult to resolve, but if such questions have not been raised about that individual's competence in other respects, then it seems unfair or inappropriate to raise them in this context.

Probably the patient did not envision the particular set of circumstances in which he or she now is in. However, that is not the point of the living will. Its point is: Is the treatment beneficial or not? Is the treatment extraordinary or not? The living will does not look at the specific circumstances of the illness but rather seeks to eliminate only one treatment option: the heroic or nonbeneficial treatment.

We assume that making some sort of disposition about one's property, money, or other affairs before death is an act of personal and social responsibility and that such decisions are binding after the individual's death. People occasionally argue over the terms of the will and how much a particular heir receives, but seldom, if ever, is the right of an individual to make such dispositions disputed. It seems reasonable to extend this line of reasoning to decisions about one's medical treatment. A person should have as much concern for his or her health needs as for money and possessions. The living will allows this concern to be actualized.

The main problem is the binding nature of the living will. The traditional last will and testament is established and supported by the legal system and is an accepted instrument for implementing one's wishes after death. Such is not the case with the living will and this raises many doubts about its value.

Legislative Responses

To resolve legal questions about a living will's binding nature, authority, and limits, many states have passed legislation validating the living will. In general such legislation has followed the sample living will developed by the Euthanasia Education Council which rejects heroic treatment. Such legislation validated the right of the person to make such a declaration and mandates that his or her wishes be followed when the person is incompetent.

There are several good reasons why such legislation should be passed.

a. Legislation would clarify the situation and one would know the status of a living will.

b. Legislation would help clarify the legal and moral obligation of a hospital and/or health care team in providing appropriate medical care.

c. Legislation would clarify who the appropriate decision-maker is. This would be particularly helpful in relieving the pressure and guilt that relatives often feel when called upon to make or participate in making such decisions.

d. Legislation would help counter the technological imperative which argues that if we can do something, we ought to do it. The living will would stop patients from being treated simply because treatment is available, even though it might be heroic.

Such arguments certainly provide strong support for current legislative efforts to enact regulations which affirm the living will and make its implementation mandatory.

On the other hand, arguments against legislation have been made which raise equally valid concerns.

a. Legislation sanctioning living wills may implicitly support the theory that the physician is the correct decision-maker and that patients have only those rights given them by specific legislation. Thus the legislation gives a wrong message.

b. Since patients already have the right to refuse treatment, legislation may undermine this situation by connoting that these rights were given by the legislature.

c. If legislation is passed, the situation of those without a living will may be worse off than it is now.

d. The legislation may be too narrowly drafted and thus fail to make allowances for the types of situations that individuals had in mind. While the intent of such legislation may be to avoid abuse, such restrictions may inhibit the legislation from functioning appropriately.

e. Legislation designed to meet all possible positions of individuals may be too difficult to draft and too cumbersome to address.

Thus the debate continues. Arguments supporting clarity and ensuring the enforceability of living wills compete with those arguing that the legislation is redundant.

Conclusions

While the arguments pro and con the living will continue, we should note that several gains have been made. There is widespread recognition that people have the right to refuse treatment. Also only a very few would argue that such a refusal constitutes evidence of incompetence. Most would hold that not everything that can be done need be done. There is a recognition that following the technological imperative leads only to a prolongation of dying, rather than to a recovery of health.

Yet many dilemmas continue to surround the decision-making process, and individuals frequently feel uncomfortable with making such serious decisions. The living will is certainly one way to approach problems such as these, for it locates the responsibility for decision-making with the patient. But since problem issues about foreseeing all circumstances or the applicability of the will to a particular illness remain, another approach is being suggested.

This approach is the designated decision-maker strategy. In such a case, you designate someone to make decisions about your health care in the event of your incompetency. The analogy for this is the power of attorney, the empowerment of one's attorney to make decisions or to execute documents on one's behalf. Applied to the health care context, one would designate an individual to be one's decision-maker. You may or may not give specific instructions about what kind of decisions to make under what kind of circumstances. But one clearly designates who is to make the decisions.

Such a solution is helpful in many ways. A decision-maker is identified. And the decision-maker is one who has agreed to perform this task. Also the solution lets the decision-maker evaluate a wide range of circumstances and be responsive to events and conditions that a living will may not have foreseen.

Whether the living will or the designated decision-maker strategy becomes the preferred solution to the problem of making decisions on behalf of incompetent patients remains to be seen. What is important is that both solutions recognize that incompetent patients have rights and that it is important to devise a strategy that allows those rights to be respected and exercised.

Topics for Discussion

1. Why has the living will become an issue?

2. Do you think that the living will may open the door to the practice of euthanasia?

3. Do you find the pro or con arguments for the living will more convincing? Why?

4. Do you think that the designated decision-maker strategy is better than the living will? Why or why not?

5. Do you think that neither strategy is necessary—that is, you think the status quo is satisfactory the way it is?

Resources

George Annas, "Rights of the Terminally Ill Patient," *Journal of Nursing Administration* 4 (March–April 1974) 40–44.
Sissela Bok, "Personal Directions for Care at the End of Life," *New England Journal of Medicine* 295 (1976) 367.

A. M. Capron, "The Development of Law on Human Death," *Annals of the New York Academy of Science* 315 (1978) 45.

Stuart J. Eisendrath and Albert R. Jonsen, "The Living Will: Help or Hindrance?" *Journal of the American Medical Association* 249 (April 15, 1983) 2054–2058.

Dennis J. Horan, "Right-to-Die Laws: Creating, Not Clarifying Problems," *Hospital Progress* 59 (June 1978) 62ff.

Luis Kunter, "Due Process of Euthanasia: The Living Will, A Proposal," *Indiana Law Journal* 44 (1969) 539.

Richard A. McCormick and Andre Hellegers, "Legislation and the Living Will," *America* 12 (March 1977).

John J. Paris and Richard A. McCormick, "Living Will Legislation, Reconsidered," *America* 145 (1981) 86.

Robert M. Veatch, "Death and Dying: The Legislative Options," *The Hastings Center Report* 7 (October 1977) 5–8.

For examples of living wills, natural death acts, and proposals for durable power of attorney, see Appendices D and E in *Deciding to Forego Life-Sustaining Treatment,* President's Commission for the Study of Ethical Problems in Medicine and Biomedical and Behavioral Research, U.S. Government Printing Office, 1983.

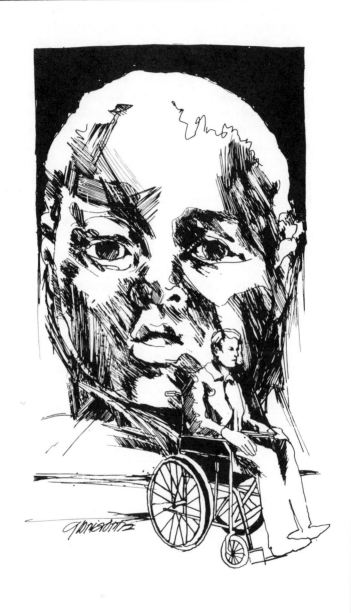

Chapter Eight

TREATMENT DECISIONS
AND NEWBORNS

Introduction

In the past several years we have been flooded with stories on newborns who are allowed to die because of physical and/or social problems they present at birth. The Bloomington Baby Doe had unconnected intestines which made oral feeding impossible. A simple surgical procedure could have easily corrected that problem but, because Baby Doe also had Down Syndrome, his parents refused the surgery. This decision was upheld by the Supreme Court of Indiana and Baby Doe died within six days of that decision.

In Illinois, a couple gave birth to Siamese twins who were incompletely formed, resulting in children with separate heads, arms, and chests, but conjoined at the pelvis and sharing a common leg. Again in this case, the parents refused surgery and requested that they not be fed. Subsequently the parents were charged with attempted homicide, but were not convicted. The babies were fed, given medical care, and they survived.

In Long Island, a couple gave birth to a child with spinal bifida. They requested treatment with medications instead of surgery. They were pursued in the courts by a right to life lawyer and the Department of Health and Human Services who thought that the child was being abused because she did not

85

receive surgery. The child survived and is home with her parents who paid a high cost to have their treatment preference validated in terms of persecution and high court costs.

These are the dramatic cases, the ones receiving national attention. But cases like these occur daily in the relative privacy of the newborn nursery. Yet these decisions are becoming more public and an increasing number of medical, ethical, and legal experts are addressing the problems that these decisions present. Also, parents appear to be more assertive in the decision-making process. There is a growing consensus that there are circumstances in which refusal or withdrawl of treatment is justified. This is most apparent in instances of severe brain damage, resulting occasionally in an almost total lack of development of the brain, multiple handicaps which prevent response to therapy, or extreme prematurity.

While not the typical outcome of birth, such tragedies happen often enough that specialized nurseries—neonatal intensive care units—have been developed and are staffed by newly trained specialists. Teams of developmental interventionists provide continual medical and developmental support of infants who are said to have "survived."

Yet these individual and team resources are frequently inadequate—for there is a limit to the support that can be given to newborns who lack critical organs or who have multiple anomalies. Often parents refuse the resources available to their child because they realize the limits of those resources in restoring their child to health, because they do not feel capable of raising such a child, or because they perceive that the child, even with the best of available medical care, will have an apparently poor or minimal quality of life. And some parents do not want a damaged child, regardless of what can be done.

Physicians and nurses will often support the decision of the parents, but they also may not. The way that information about the child is presented can determine how the parents decide. Value judgments are continually being made, but frequently under the guise of hospital policy or medical judgment. These decisions seem to be easier to make when they are described as something other than what they actually are: value judgments or quality of life judgments.

Whatever the type of judgment, however, more and more people seem to be deciding to forego treating their newborns in the hope that they will die quietly and mercifully.

The response to this is varied, of course. Some individuals have very cogently argued that such a practice is severe neglect of physicians' and parents' obligation to provide a minimal standard of care for those for whom they are responsible. Such neglect of duty—evidenced by refusing appropriate medical treatment or food which results in death—is homicide.[1] Others argue that in justice all infants must be treated equally unless there is some morally relevant difference between them. If two infants are born with the problem of a blocked intestine but the second one also has Down Syndrome, many would argue that justice is violated if only the former is treated. Others argue that the quality of the infant's life must be evaluated and decisions about treatment be made on the basis of what kind of quality could be expected. Finally, some argue that all life is valuable and must be preserved regardless of circumstances or quality.

Thus the issues are joined: right to life vs. quality of life; duty to care vs. feelings of inadequacy; technical ability to maintain vs. responsibility for long term care; medical prognosis vs. value judgments; hospital policy vs. parental decisions; law vs. conscience.

These are but a sampling of the dilemmas raised by thinking about the decisions to be made on behalf of newborns with various problems. Several of these issues will be considered, as well as discussing the latest federal regulations on the treatment of infants.

Elements in the Discussion

Medical
Two developments need discussion here, the diagnostic and the technical. The diagnostic procedure of amniocentesis per-

mits the prenatal diagnosis of several hundred genetic diseases, as well as identifying the sex of the fetus. A needle is inserted through the mother's abdomen into the uterus and collects the amnionic fluid which contains fetal cells. These cells are then cultured and their genetic status examined. Although a disease can be diagnosed, at present there is no way to treat the disease. Consequently the response to a diagnosis may be an abortion.

Two perspectives are debated in this context. First, curing or preventing a disease by killing the patient is typically not the way medicine conducts its business. But abortions are done in response to learning of the diagnosis of a genetic disease. This is why many in the right to life movement refer to amniocentesis as a "search and destroy" mission. The other perspective is that amniocentesis may save lives by ensuring that only fetuses with genetic diseases are aborted. Parents who know only the probability of the fetus' actually being affected may abort a healthy fetus. Thus by determining whether the fetus is actually affected, amniocentesis can save fetal lives.

The technical element in the debate is the neonatal intensive care unit. New technologies permit better monitoring, more access, and better support of the newborn. Developments in technology are complemented by the growing knowledge and skills of the neonatologists. Such increases in care and support systems have allowed fetuses as young as twenty or twenty-one weeks old to survive outside the uterus.

Such successes are also complemented with the ongoing problems of high tech medicine alluded to elsewhere in this book. The same issues of allocation of resources, decisions of withholding or withdrawing treatment, costs, and quality of life affect the newborn nursery as well as other areas of health care. Thus while tremendous accomplishments have been made, other dilemmas continue to present themselves.

The context
The pediatric relationship is one of the more complex ones in medicine. There are at least four main actors: the infant, the physician, the parents, and society. I will comment on each.

The infant is a separate, living member of the human species and as such has significant moral value. But the infant is helpless, incompetent, and has no experience of his or her condition or sense of what it might mean. The infant has a future but no past. Consequently issues of the infant's best interest arise, determinations about its quality of life are sought, and questions of long term support are raised. While the infant is valued, questions of how that value can be actualized are raised.

The physician is a professional with a certain level of training and his or her own standard of professional ethics. The physician also has a range of experience and can make reasonable judgments about the future of the infant. The physician also has his or her personal standards by which the infant is experienced and evaluated.

The parents have their hopes and expectations, their values, their standards. Typically they experience guilt, anxiety, and fear because of the condition of their child. Their reality is severely disturbed because the child of their dreams is not the child they experience. But nonetheless they are the parents and have responsibility for the child.

Finally, society in the form of hospital policy, state and federal law, religion, or the court can enter into the relation. Hospital policy, following state and federal law, may state a particular standard of care to which it will hold physician and parents. Court cases and/or regulations may shape how an infant is or is not treated. In each instance, the parents and physicians are not autonomous actors, but operate within the social fabric which has an effect on how they act.

All of these elements serve to complicate further an already complex situation and sharpen any conflict that may be in the situation. But, clearly, the multifaceted dimensions of the relationship require special care in articulating the issues.

Decision-making

There are two major issues in decision-making: Who should make the decision, and on what basis?

1. Who decides? Several decision-makers have been proposed. First, the parents. They are the ones who wanted the child.
They are the ones who will experience the impact of raising the
child, and they are the ones who have responsibility for the
child. Historically, parents have been charged with making
decisions for their children, and society assumes that, absent
evidence to the contrary, parents typically decide in the best
interests of the child.

Physicians are also proposed as decision-makers. They
have skill and experience in dealing with these cases. They have
professional standards of care to uphold and they are committed
to preserving life. But it is the physicians' medical expertise
that most often commends them as decision makers.

Others suggest that society in the form of the court of law be
the decision-maker. The hope is that these methods would be
more objective and, therefore, give a fairer decision. The other
purpose of having society involved is so that the decision-
making process will be in the open and that a certain amount of
consistency will be obtained.

Finally, ethics committees have been suggested as appropriate decision-makers. Such committees would explicitly deal
with the value dimensions of such cases. Thus the decisions
would not be hidden under the guise of medical or technical
decisions. While an ethics committee would help surface the
ethical aspects of a case, questions of its competence, authority
and scope are still being debated.

2. On what basis? Typically, three standards are suggested
as the basis of decision-making. First is a medical basis. The
primary issues here are: Is the condition treatable? Is it
manageable? Is it reversible? Can the patient be benefitted
medically? Value judgments about best interest or quality of life
are essentially discarded in favor of a determination of whether
or not an intervention is possible and will medically benefit the
child.

A second set of standards revolve around the issue of the
quality of life orientation. This is an attempt to recognize that
while physical life is a value, it may not be the ultimate value.

There are two standard ways of articulating this orientation. First is the best interests standard. Decisions are made on the basis of what appears to be best overall for the child. Here one would include medical elements, but would also evaluate socio-economic issues, the potential of the child, the resources available for long term care, and the sort of future the child may have.

The second is the substituted judgment standard. Here one tries to situate oneself in the position of the child and then make the decision you think the individual would make if he or she knew what you know. The attempt here is to factor into the decision relevant information, but to avoid arbitrariness. One tries to determine what decision the patient would make if the patient were aware of the situation, and then use that as the actual decision.

Finally, one would rely on the traditional ordinary/extra-ordinary standard as the basis for the decision. Here one could take into account a future of severe pain, continued serious and extremely burdensome medical or surgical procedures, or the futility of a particular therapy with respect to its ability to restore the patient to a reasonable standard of health.

Legal issues

Two critical legal issues present themselves. First, is the withholding of treatment a violation of the physician's and parents' duty to care? Typically, the helpless condition of a child places strong obligations on parents and physicians to provide support, the necessities of life, and the medical care necessary to preserve the child's life. Failure to do so leading to the child's death has typically been seen as criminal homicide by omission. While some have seen the circumstances of the intensive care unit as carving out an exception to this, others have argued that the standard of care is the same in all circumstances.

The second legal issue is that of discrimination against the handicapped by withholding or withdrawing treatment. The issue is: If the infant did not have these handicaps, would treatment be denied? This is an especially relevant question when mental retardation is also part of the clinical picture. Our cultural values and social expectations frequently shape how we evaluate an individual. This orientation seeks to retain a degree of objectivity by eliminating prejudicial elements from decision-making.

Ethical issues

All decisions made on behalf of incompetent individuals are paternalistic.[2] That is, they are either made on someone's behalf but not at that person's request, or they are refusals to cooperate with another's wishes. These decisions are also acts of hard paternalism in that of necessity they involve the value system of someone other than the patient. They are also direct in that the person on whose behalf the decision is made experiences the consequences of that decision. In situations such as these it is important to remember that the decisions made should be the least restrictive, beneficial, and the least insulting to the potential freedom of the individual.

Beneficence, the duty to do good to others, is also important in this context. Clearly the patient has a problem, may be in pain, and has the needs associated with helplessness. If anyone has a claim to beneficent actions, surely it is the individual who is sick and helpless.

The discussion about ordinary and extraordinary means of treatment is relevant to this discussion, remembering of course the qualifications placed on this distinction in earlier chapters. One needs to examine carefully the treatment and its impact upon the infant and his or her condition. One also needs to establish, within reasonable medical judgment, whether the treatment is prolonging dying or having a beneficial effect.

The final ethical issue is the debate between the right to life and the quality of life. The right to life position argues that life is the most important value, and that if that value is not protected and defended against assaults, then all else stands to be lost. When human life loses its value, then other institutions and values are also endangered. The value of life and the dignity of the person stand at the center of the moral and cultural universe, and if they are degraded or disregarded, we have lost our moral foundation.

But the quality of life is important also. How people live or the conditions under which they live is often more important than whether they live. The defense of the values of democracy and liberty as well as human dignity itself in war is surely an example of some values sometimes being as or more important than life itself. Also, if one looks at the history of moral theology, one finds examples of quality of life arguments being used. The development of the doctrine of the just war is one. So is the acceptance of the practice of taking interest on loans. An almost total prohibition on usury was rejected by the Catholic Church so that capital could be put into the economy to help social growth. The right of the employer to profits was qualified by the workers' right to a just wage. And procreation can be limited, with the use of certain means, for medical, economic, or educational reasons.

Both the right to life and the quality of life have strong arguments on their side. Perhaps each should be seen as a corrective on the other so that an uncritical application of either can be avoided.

The State of the Question

Because of the stormy nature of the debate over the treatment of newborns, the highly visible media attention given to these cases, and the level of professional and lay concerns about the issue, federal regulations about the treatment of newborns were proposed. I will present an overview of these regulations and comment on their significance.

The main features of the regulations are the definitions of medical neglect and the withholding of treatment. Medical neglect is defined as including, but "not limited to, the withholding of medically indicated treatment from a disabled infant with a life-threatening condition."[3] The term "withholding of medically indicated treatment" means "the failure to respond to the infant's life-threatening conditions by providing treatment (including appropriate nutrition, hydration, and medication) which, in the treating physician's (or physicians') reasonable medical judgment, will be most likely to be effective in ameliorating or correcting all such conditions."[4]

These definitions provide critical clarifications. As far as federal regulations were concerned, failure to provide appropriate treatment would be illegal. Also the withholding of food and water, even though administered only intravenously, constitutes medical neglect and is prohibited. These two elements would resolve, at least on a regulatory level, many of the debates.

Included in the definition of withholding treatment are three exceptions, again based on reasonable medical judgment.

1. The infant is chronically and irreversibly comatose.

2. The provision of such treatment would merely prolong dying, not be effective in ameliorating or correcting all of the infant's life-threatening conditions, or otherwise be futile in terms of the survival of the infant.

3. The providing of such treatment would be virtually futile in terms of the survival of the infant, and the treatment itself under such circumstances would be inhumane.[5]

Most importantly, the withholding of appropriate nutrition, hydration, or medication is excluded from these exceptions. That is, even though the regulations provide for the withholding of therapy from an infant, and this particular infant qualifies for such a withholding of therapy, food, water and medication may not be withheld. This regulation clearly prohibits the practice of not feeding infants from whom treatment is withheld.

As such, these definitions and regulations speak clearly and firmly to the debates and practice concerning infants with birth anomalies. They also reflect a clear value orientation. The ethical framework used to resolve the debate most closely resembles the medical indications policy described above. That is, the criterion for determining what to do is whether, in reasonable medical judgment, there is a treatment that will benefit the infant. The test is medical, and, consequently, the decision-maker is the physician.

Also the regulations suggest that Infant Care Review Committees may be established. The regulations do not mandate such committees, but advisory guidelines are provided for those who wish to do so. Of interest is the name and the suggested membership of such a committee. The purpose of the committee is to review the care of the infant—hence its title. Absent is an identification of the committee as an ethics committee. Also the suggested membership consists of a physician, nurse, hospital administrator, a social worker, a representative of a disability group, a lay member, and a member of the medical staff who will serve as the chair. Conspicuous by absence is someone with expertise in ethics.

The absence of ethics in the committee title and from membership on the committee is explained in the commentary of the guidelines. "The Department [of Health and Human Services] has not changed the title of the committee because nothing in the authorizing statute corroborates the notion that the focus of the committee should be 'medical ethics,' at least to the extent that term connotes considerations different than those involved in evaluating medical treatment possibilities that 'will be most likely to be effective in ameliorating or correcting' all life-threatening conditions."6 Thus the only decision to be made is the medical appropriateness of the treatment, and any review committee is charged only with the review of that. Clearly this review eliminates considerations of quality of life, prohibits the withholding of food, water, and medication, and makes the physician the decision-maker.

The resolution of these issues provided by the proposed regulations was upset by the Supreme Court. On June 9, 1986 the Court ruled by a 4 to 3 majority that there was no evidence that handicapped babies had been discriminated against by hospitals. Thus there was no need for the regulations. Consequently the debate is again open.

Notes

1. John Robertson, "Involuntary Euthanasia of Defective Newborns: A Legal Analysis," *Stanford Law Review* 27, 213ff.

2. For a fuller discussion of paternalism, confer James Childress, *Who Shall Decide? Paternalism in Health Care.* Oxford University Press, 1982.

3. *The Federal Register,* Vol. 50, No. 72, April 15, 1985, 14887.

4. *Ibid.,* 14888.

5. *Ibid.*

6. *Ibid.,* 14897.

Topics for Discussion

1. If you were pregnant and your physician recommended amniocentesis, what would be your reaction? Would having an amniocentesis raise any moral questions for you?

2. Whom do you think the decision-maker ought to be?

3. What should be the basis of the decision?

4. Should quality of life issues play any role in the decision-making process?

5. What is your feeling about the proposed federal regulations?

Bibliography

American Academy of Pediatrics, "Treatment of Critically Ill Newborns," *Pediatrics,* Vol. 72, No. 4 (October 1983) 565.

Department of Health and Human Services, "Child Abuse and Neglect Prevention and Treatment Program," *Federal Register* 50 (April 15, 1985) 14878–14901.

Raymond Duff, M.D., "Counseling Families and Deciding Care of Severely Defective Children: A Way of Coping With 'Medical Vietnam,'" *Pediatrics,* Vol. 67, No. 3 (March 1981) 315.

Alan R. Fleischman and Thomas H. Murray, "Ethics Committees for Infants Doe," *The Hastings Center Report* (December 1983) 5.

Norman Fost, "Counseling Families Who Have a Child with a Severe Congenital Anomaly," *Pediatrics,* Vol. 67, No. 3 (March 1981) 321.

Michael L. Hardman and Clifford J. Drew, "Parental Consent and the Practice of Withholding Treatment from the Severely Defective Newborn," *Mental Retardation* (August 1980) 165.

Albert R. Jonsen, "The Ethics of Pediatric Medicine," *Pediatrics,* A. M. Rudolph and J. I. Hoffman, editors. Appleton Century Croft, 1982 (17th Edition) 9–18.

Thomas H. Murray, "The Final, Anticlimactic Rule on Baby Doe," *The Hastings Center Report* (June 1985) 5.

Thomas A. Shannon and Paula R. Rosen, "Chad Green: Dilemmas in Legal and Ethical Decision Making," *New Physician* (February 1981) 35 and 38.

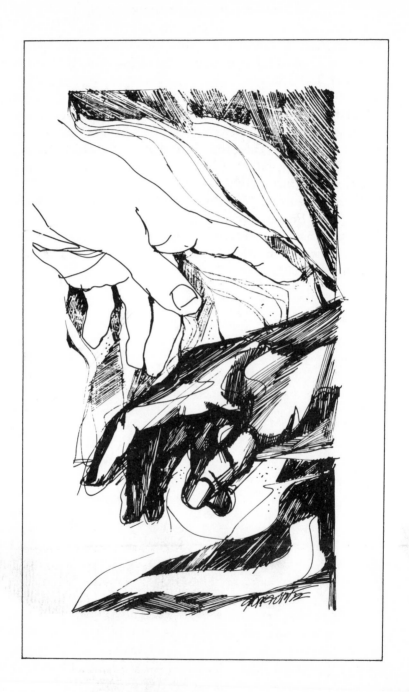

Chapter Nine

ORGAN TRANSPLANTS

Introduction

If there is one area in modern medicine where many break-throughs and exciting developments have occurred, it is the area of organ transplants. While we have not achieved the feats associated with the six million dollar man and the bionic woman, nonetheless new developments in drug therapies, transplantation procedures, and the development of a variety of new artificial organs have changed how we think of organ transplantation.

A story in the New York *Times*[1] listed a variety of companies and the bionic replacements they manufacture: ears, wrists, knees, legs or arms, ankles, blood vessels, toe joints, shoulder and knee ligaments, shoulders, elbows, hips, and lens implants. Of course, we must add to this the artificial heart which has been used on several patients, as either a permanent or a temporary replacement. Organ transplantations continue and the drug cyclosporin has helped decrease the rejection of these transplanted organs.

Yet, some problems persist. The demand for organs continues to outstrip the supply, as has been dramatized nationally in well conducted media assisted searches for organs. The boundaries between research and therapy are occasionally blurred.

Issues of allocation of resources continue to be raised as costs of dialysis and transplantation continue to mount.

In this chapter, I will review several background issues, ethical issues, and then discuss the artificial heart.

Background Issues

Technical

Several technical issues present themselves. First, research continues to develop materials which will not harm the blood or other organic substances against which the device or artificial organ comes in contact. The material must be able, for example, both to prevent blood from clotting and also not to destroy the blood cells. And as mentioned, research continues on drugs which will suppress the immune system of the recipient so that his or her body will not reject the organ. Needed is a balance between a drug strong enough to prevent rejection but not so strong that the body will be defenseless against infections. Finally, there is a need to develop a more appropriate power source for the artificial heart. While advances have been made, the power source is still external and requires another individual to transport it.

General

Other issues are somewhat more difficult to categorize. They are social in nature, are pre-ethical, and have to do with the nature of the medical establishment. For example, would the money spent on the development and use of artificial organs be better spent on educational efforts for prevention? Should medical practice be shifted from attempts to cure disease to attempts to prevent it in the first place? Such a shift would dramatically alter the way medicine is understood and would have a significant impact on the next two generations. Yet such a shift would clearly be cheaper in the long run.

Second, at the present time kidney dialysis is essentially subsidized by the federal government. The cost for this is over a billion dollars annually and costs will continue to rise. Should other diseases be subsidized in the same or a similar fashion? Why does dialysis have this privileged position? It is very clear that if other catastrophic diseases were treated in the same or similar way, the entire federal budget would be devoted to health care. Efforts need to be made to plan the future of health subsidies in our country.

Third, should private behavior be modified in the interest of prevention or the public good? For example, if people did not smoke cigarettes, lung cancer rates would decrease dramatically. If people did not live the life style associated with the pursuit and use of illegal drugs, many deaths and illnesses would be prevented. If pregnant women eat properly and do not smoke or drink, the probability of a premature birth decreases. If people wear seat belts, car accident fatalities decrease. And so on, and so on. Such regulation of individual behavior is typically disapproved of—witness the public outcry over legislation mandating the use of helmets while riding motorcycles and requiring the wearing of seat belts. The tension between individual freedom and the public good is raised sharply here.

The issues standing behind concerns such as these is one of priorities. What should be our goals in medicine? What strategies should we adopt in pursuing these goals? How far can individual life styles be regulated? And what is the role of the federal government in both setting goals and subsidizing the strategies to achieve them? Until these issues are debated and resolved, many of the dilemmas surrounding organ transplantation will not be easily resolved.

Ethical Issues

Justification of transplantation

There are two ways to think about the issues involved in transplantation. The first involves the justification of one person, while living, giving an organ to another. In so doing, the donor violates the integrity of his or her body and puts himself or herself at some risk from both the surgery and possible future health complications. On the other hand, many organs come in pairs and we can function as well with only one. The kidney is a prime example of this. In this light, the justification for such a donation is threefold: (1) the duty of beneficence which requires us to do good to others when the risk to ourselves is reasonable; (2) the good to be realized by the recipient in terms of increased life span and quality of life; (3) the modest risks undertaken by the donor.

A second way of justification was proposed by James Nelson. He identified five principles that are still valid as a means of evaluating a particular transplantation. (1) The transplantation is the last resort. No other remedies are possible and what is available has failed. (2) The primary intent is the patient's welfare. This is to ensure that the primary concern is clinical, not experimental. (3) Consent to the procedure must be free and informed. The patient must know the risks, the benefits, the other options, and must give permission for the procedure. (4) The protection of the innocent. Nelson's point is that all involved—the patient, family members, and the donor—must not be given false hopes, the rights of the patient must be respected, and the donor—especially one likely to be declared brain dead—must be protected. (5) Proportionality. The benefits of the procedure must outweigh the risks or the costs. While having a quality of life dimension to it, this criterion also looks to questions of medical feasibility.

How do we obtain organs?

The traditional way organs have been obtained is by donation, or more formally, through the principle of voluntariness. This principle ensured that the donor's consent would be obtained and that he or she would be free of coercion. The hope was that such voluntarism, expressed through mechanisms such as a direct gift, a donor card, an affirmation on a driver's license, or through a provision in a living will, would provide enough organs. Such was not the case, and the demand far outstrips the supply.

New strategies to obtain organs have come forward. One is a massive education program. Such efforts have been tried in the past but have not been that successful. Another is the free market approach in which individuals will sell their organs at whatever price the market will bear. Although clearly in the grand tradition of free enterprise, most commentators have found the sale of body parts to be ethically repulsive since they imply an objectification of the body and a violation of human dignity, and they open the way to coercive practices. A third suggestion is to establish legislation which says that if one has not stated that he or she does not want to be a donor, then at death the state owns the body and can harvest any usable organs. Thus if one wished not to be a donor, one would have to explicitly state this; otherwise the organs would be taken. While this proposal makes provision for choice and would greatly increase the supply of organs, others feel that this proposal devalues the cadaver to too great an extent. By making it a commodity immediately upon death, the memory of the person who was present through it can be violated and the feelings of the survivors can be offended. A final proposal attempts a compromise. A law first in New York and now in many states it requires that the family of a patient who is dying or has died be asked if that individual's organs can be used. This "required request," as Arthur Caplan calls it,[3] protects voluntariness, provides the family with the opportunity to exercise beneficence establishes a practice that all will come to expect, and directly addresses the reason why many families do not donate organs: they are not asked. New York's pioneering legislation will be important to watch to determine whether the supply of organs is increased and whether or not families feel ethically offended by such a request.

Patient Selection
In 1985, the Massachusetts Task Force on Organ Transplantation issued a report that included, among other items, a discussion of methods of patient selection.[4] The values upon which a selection system should be based are fairness, efficiency, the value of life, and other important social values.

Schemes of selection that typically have been proposed, and which should be reviewed in the light of these values, include, first, the market approach. Here organs can be obtained by those who can pay for them either through their own capital or through a private insurance plan. Such a plan obviously violates equity.

Second is the committee approach. In the early days of dialysis, such an approach was used but eventually rejected. It became apparent that the committee was explicitly using social status criteria as the basis of their decisions. Such arbitrariness, whether conscious or unconscious, disregarded the value of life and totally rejected fairness.

The lottery approach, whether of the first come, first served type or the pull the number out of the hat type, attempts to be equitable by giving all in need an equal chance. Yet such a system may not be efficient or fair because it equates those with a better long term prognosis with those without such a prognosis.

Fourth, the Task Force identifies the customary approach. This is descriptive, in that it reports what people do. In England, for example, it has been customary not to give dialysis to individuals over fifty-five. This practice was neither well known nor publicly decided upon. Increases in end stage renal disease may result in unnecessary death, and the policy may be forced to change because of the valuing of life over money. In the United States, clinical suitability is frequently the criterion referred to. However, this standard may contain hidden agenda such as the typical requirement of a family to provide a support network. As the report notes about the customary approach: "It gives us the illusion that we don't have to make choices; but the cost is deception, and when this deception is uncovered, we must deal with it either by universal entitlement or by choosing another method of patient selection."[5]

The task force proposed a combination approach. First there must be an initial screening based exclusively on medical criteria, including length of survival and capacity for rehabilitation. Also there should be sensitivity to the fact that the poor frequently are worse off medically because of their poverty. Thus medical criteria should be fair and public.

After this pool of applicants is developed, the Task Force recommends a first come, first served lottery, with one exception. Individuals can advance if the second level review committee thinks the individual is in danger of death and the candidate originally scheduled can live long enough to be assured that he or she will obtain an organ.

Criteria such as these will not resolve all problems—increased demand, fewer organs, higher costs—but they put a degree of fairness into the system and eliminate to a large degree arbitrariness and social worth judgments.

What is the price of life?

The issue of resource allocation, whether in terms of the organs themselves, the staff and facilities for the transplant and follow-up care, or the funding of transplantations, ultimately may be the key issue. Regardless of how much we value life, how dearly we hold to life, or how central the right to life is in our value scheme, ultimately a price tag is attached and someone must pay.

These costs include, but are not limited to, dialysis, whether temporary or long term, hospitalization, follow up care, supplies, medication, physical and dietary therapy, and the storage and transplantation of organs. When, for example in 1982 there were more than 65,000 individuals receiving dialysis, one can appreciate that the cost is exceptionally high. The projected Medicare costs for the estimated 90,000 patients in 1995 is $5.5 billion. The 1982 costs are almost $2 billion.

While it is a truism that there is a lot of fat in all budgets, it remains a fact that one can rob Peter to pay Paul only so long. All budgets are finite, and regardless of the degree of creativity in shifting budget lines or improvising new accounts, ultimately there is only so much money to spend. Our society has been typically reluctant to face such a brutal reality. Thus a major task of the next decade will be to resolve the tension between the value of life and the price of life.

The Artificial Heart

Developments in and the use of the artificial heart have given rise to several reactions. First, the symbolic. The heart is the symbol of a human's deepest emotions, and even though we know it is also a pump, replacing a biological heart with a mechanical one raises profound emotional issues. Second, since the heart, along with the brain, is responsible for keeping individuals alive, removing it is exceptionally risky. Even though the individual faces certain death because of his or her illness, removing the heart guarantees death—absent a transplant or a mechanical heart. Research on the artificial heart has raised again the question of whether prevention or cure of heart disease is more important. Would money be better spent on education or research? How does one die when one has an artificial heart? Does one experience multiple system failure, such as Dr. Barney Clark, did? Does one negotiate the turning off of the power system. Does one rely on brain death exclusively as the preferred definition of death?

These and other questions have been vigorously debated since 1957 when the artificial heart program began. In 1960, the first artificial heart was implanted in a dog that lived for ninety minutes. In 1963, the National Heart Institute began an artificial heart program and federal funding began in 1964. The program did not develop as quickly as hoped and other devices were developed to assist the heart. Then in 1969, Dr. Denton Cooly implanted the first artificial heart in a human to be used until an organic heart could be found. Research continued, funded both federally and privately (160 million federal dollars by 1983), and on December 2, 1982 Dr. William DeVries implanted a newly developed artificial heart into Dr. Barney Clark who lived for 112 days after the operation. A total of six transplants have occurred as of this writing.

Much has been learned about the design of the heart, the external power source has been reduced considerably, and the glare of publicity and the minute by minute press conferences have decreased. However some problems remain. Bleeding continues to be an issue as well as fear of infections. But the major problem is blood clotting and the consequent threat or actuality of strokes. The cause of the clotting is unclear which is hampering efforts to remedy it.

A national panel, commissioned after the recent wave of publicity about and re-examination of the new efforts, recommended that federal efforts to develop a totally implantable permanent artificial heart be expanded. The commission stated that such a device could "provide a significant increase in life span, with an acceptable quality of life, for 17,000 to 35,000 patients below age 70 annually."[6] The commission also estimated that the implant would cost about $150,000 and that recipients would survive an average of four and a half years.

Clearly the implantation of the artificial heart has raised the hopes of those with incurable heart disease and with little or no hope of obtaining a transplantation. The artificial heart gives these individuals one last hope. Yet questions of quality of life remain. Confinement, low levels of activity, risk of stroke, and media attention all may have a profound impact on how one lives.

Many questions need to be answered and many problems remain, but both research and practice are going forward. Careful monitoring and analysis of the results will help us to better evaluate this significant development.

Notes

1. The New York *Times,* November 20, 1983, Section 3, p. 1.

2. James Nelson, *Human Medicine.* Augsburg Publishing House, 1973, pp. 152ff.

3. Arthur L. Caplan. "Ethical and Policy Issues in the Procurement of Cadaver Organs for Transplantation," *The New England Journal of Medicine,* Vol. 313, No. 15, p. 938.

4. "Report of the Massachusetts Task Force on Organ

Transplantation," *Law, Medicine, and Health Care,* Vol. 13, No. 1, pp. 8–26.

5. *Ibid.,* p. 19.

6. Lawrence K. Altman, "U.S. Panel Gives Heart Implant Firm Backing," The New York *Times,* May 24, 1985, p. 1.

Discussion Questions

1. Do you have any objections to the transplantation of organs?

2. What do you think is a fair system of allocating the available organs?

3. What do you think is a responsible way of obtaining organs?

4. Do you think the artificial heart is a good idea? Should research continue on it?

5. Do you think that organs should be transplanted from animals to humans, as in the Baby Fae case?

Bibliography

Arthur L. Caplan, "Ethical and Policy Issues in the Procurement of Cadaver Organs for Transplantation," *The New England Journal of Medicine,* Vol. 131, No. 15, pp. 981ff.

William C. DeVries *et al.,* "Clinical Use of the Total Artificial Heart," *The New England Journal of Medicine,* Vol. 310, No. 5, p. 274.

Renee Fox and Judith Swazey, *The Courage to Fail: A Social View of Organ Transplants and Dialysis.* The University of Chicago Press, 1974.

John K. Inglehart. "Transplantation: The Problem of Limited Resources," *The New England Journal of Medicine,* Vol. 309, No. 2, p. 123.

Jay Katz and Alexander M. Capron, *Catastrophic Diseases: Who Decides What?* Russell Sage Foundation, 1975.

Report of the Massachusetts Task Force on Organ Transplantation," *Law, Medicine and Health Care,* Vol. 13, No. 1, p. 8.

Richard Titmuss, *The Gift Relationship: From Human Blood to Social Policy.* Pantheon Books, 1970.

F. Ross Woolley, "Ethical Issues in the Implantation of the Artificial Heart," *The New England Journal of Medicine,* Vol. 310, No. 5, p. 292.

Stuart J. Younger *et al.,* "Psychosocial and Ethical Implications of Organ Retrieval," *The New England Journal of Medicine,* Vol. 313, No. 5, p. 321.

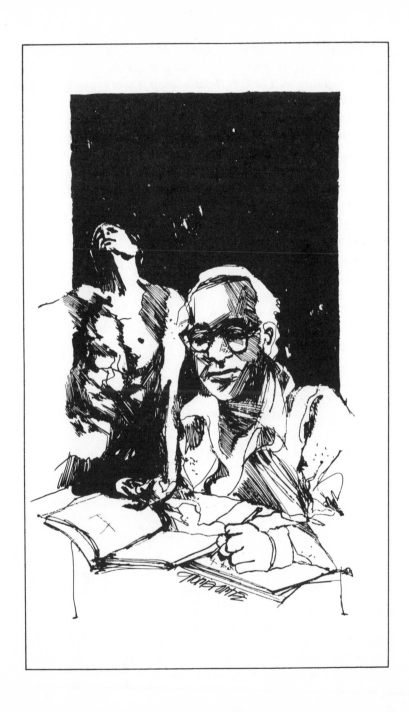

Chapter Ten

RESEARCH ON
HUMAN SUBJECTS

Introduction

Although most of the work of the work of medical researchers is carried out in the laboratory, unknown and unobserved by the public, probably no feature of modern medicine has had as dramatic an effect on as many people as research. By careful design and countless hours of running experiments, scientists have succeeded in identifying the causes of many diseases and have designed vaccines to prevent them. The elimination of smallpox, most childhood diseases, and other sources of human illness have been eliminated because of research into their causes. These same efforts are being marshaled against the major diseases of our day: cancer, AIDS, and heart disease.

Yet while having all these benefits, some problems have been associated with research, especially in the last several decades. Several well publicized cases involving the involuntary infection of children with hepatitis, injecting live cancer cells into nursing home residents, and not treating diagnosed syphilis so that the natural course of the disease could be observed raised problems about consent. The experiments conducted by Nazi physicians in the concentration camps raised questions about the motives of the physicians and the value of the knowledge gained. And more recently publicized cases of fraud through data faking either by inventing patients or by manufacturing experiments focused on the dangers of a too highly competitive atmosphere in the lab.

Concerns such as these as well as the desire to ensure the traditionally high standards of research and the integrity of the scientists led to a long national process of examining the ethics of research on human subjects. This chapter will highlight some of the elements of that process.

Ethical Issues in Research on Human Subjects

Consent

The key issue in research is consent. Consent, first, protects the patient's autonomy. By consenting (or not consenting) to the research, the patient has assumed control over his or her life. Second, consent protects human dignity. The patient is recognized as a center of value who cannot be used as an object. Third, consent is functional in that it reassures the public that they are not being manipulated or deceived. Fourth, consent promotes trust between subject and physician. Finally, consent can help the subject become a better subject. By knowing more of the research project, the subject can perhaps provide better information, be more cooperative, and especially be more diligent in fulfilling the requirements of the study. This last element is especially important in studies which can last several months or even years. Thus for both ethical and practical reasons consent is important.

Selection of Subjects

In an older but still classic article, Hans Jonas defined four categories of possible research subjects.[1]

1. The best educated, most highly motivated members of society, typically represented by the researcher-scientists. The tradition of self-experimentation has had an honored place in science and many researchers still participate in the research protocol, at least to know what the subjects are experiencing.

2. The most marginal people in society: the defenseless, the poor, the powerless. These people would not be able to resist the power of the scientific establishment, and they ensure a type of captive audience.

3. Those willing to sell their services. This method of recruitment is in the spirit of free enterprise so valued by our American society. The only issue is that the price be right.

4. Conscription by lottery from the public at large. Since all have benefited from advances in medicine, all repay this benefit by participating in research. Also this is a type of public service that could demonstrate one's civic responsibilities. Although never used before, it is a fair way to obtain subjects.

There is another way of obtaining subjects, which is probably the most typical. Physicians frequently ask their patients to participate in research by trying a new drug, a new procedure, or a new device. While this option provides the possibility of a direct benefit to the subject as well as advances in knowledge, it has the disadvantage of blurring the roles of physician and researcher and between clinical practice and research.

The issue behind all of these schemes is fairness. The concern is to ensure that no one population is singled out for continual use in research or is in some way put at risk because of an inability to resist requests to participate.

The Obligation to Participate in Research

The issue of fairness in obtaining subjects forces us to ask the question about whether there might be an obligation to participate in research. Some have suggested that a sense of fair play would require that all be willing to participate in research. Since I have benefited from others who have been research subjects, I should participate so that others can benefit.

Altruism also can be a motivation for participation in research. Altruism focuses on the benefits to society and the good to be received by those in need. Such generosity of spirit could motivate others willingly to participate and can help create bonds of community between the ill and the healthy.

Another justification for research stresses the utilitarian

orientation. People are obligated to participate in research because of the benefits gained by society and because of the valuable knowledge that can be attained.

All of these orientations provide a decent justification for participating in research. And since our system of recruitment is primarily based on voluntarism, each must evaluate and determine his or her sense of an obligation to participate in research if asked.

The Public Conducting of Research

Because of the publicity given to problems in the conducting of research, some of which were alluded to in the opening paragraphs, a rather lengthy public discussion of how research was conducted was held. The primary forums for this debate were a presidential commission, discussion by the Department of Health and Human Services, and the eventual development of federal regulations.[2]

One result of these discussions was the creation of a set of federal regulations on how human research ought to be conducted (45 Code of Federal Regulations 46). These regulations do two primary things. First, they clearly define informed consent: the knowing consent of an individual or his or her legally authorized representative, so situated as to be able to exercise free power of choice, without undue inducement or any element of force, fraud, deceit, duress, or other form of constraint or cooercion. While this standard is rather high, it highlights the value of autonomy and sets the standard high to protect the value.

Second, the regulations spell out the information that must be given.

1. An explanation of the procedures and their purposes, making sure the subject knows that they are experimental.
2. Identifying the risks and discomforts that can be reasonably expected.
3. A description of possible benefits.

4. An indication of alternative therapies available.
5. An offer to answer any questions the subject has.
6. Affirming that the subject may withdraw from the experiment at any time without penalty.

The means by which these regulations are implemented is the Institutional Review Board (IRB). The IRB is not explicitly established by the regulations, but its existence is certainly presumed by it. Thus many commentators assume that the authority of the IRB comes from the institution which it represents and has as much (or as little) power as the institution gives it. An IRB can do human research only mandated by federal regulation or it can review all research on humans performed in the institution.

The IRB's tasks are basically twofold. First, the IRB reviews and monitors research conducted at its institution. Second, it evaluates the balance between risk and benefit in particular protocols. The purpose of this is to ensure the intelligibility of the protocol and to discuss and determine the acceptability of the risk benefit ratio. This review attempts to assure that the autonomy of the patient is protected.

While IRBs do add another layer of bureaucracy and paperwork between the research and the investigator, research appears to continue at its normal pace. Rather than reject proposals, most IRBs seem to prefer to resolve differences by negotiation. Sometimes, as in the case of the first use of the artificial heart, these negotiations are lengthy and sometimes, as in the case of the first transplantation of an animal heart into a human, they are highly criticized. Nonetheless, the system appears to be working well and has provided another means of protecting subjects, without disrupting the research enterprise.

Notes

1. Hans Jonas, "Philosophical Reflections on Experimenting with Human Subjects," *Daedalus,* Spring 1969, p. 219.
2. 45 CFR 46: 103.

Questions for Discussion

1. Why is consent so important in research?
2. How do you think research subjects should be recruited or selected?
3. Would you participate in a research experiment?
4. Do you think research subjects should be paid for participating in research? Should they pay for tests, medications, or other costs such as travel or should these be provided?
5. Pregnant women are typically excluded from research projects. This means that when a new drug is released, no one knows the effect of the drug on the fetus. Can you think of an ethical way to resolve this problem?

Bibliography

George Annas, Leonard Glanz, and Barbara Katz, *Informed Consent to Human Experimentation: The Subject's Dilemma.* The Ballinger Publishing Company, 1977.

Henry K. Beecher, *Research in the Individual: Human Studies.* Little and Brown, Inc., 1970.

Karen Lebacqz and Robert J. Levine, "Respect for Persons and Informed Consent To Participate in Research," *Clinical Research 27: 101–107.*

Robert J. Levine. "The Impact of Institutional Review Boards on Clinical Research," *Perspectives in Biology and Medicine,* Winter 1980, p. 98.

———. *Ethics and Regulation of Clinical Research.* Urban and Schwarzenberg, 1981.

President's Commission for the Study of Ethical Problems in Medicine and Biomedical and Behavioral Research, *Compensation for Research Injuries,* U.S. Government Printing Office, 1982.

Alice Rivlin and P. Michael Timpane, Editors, *Ethical and Legal Issues of Social Experimentation.* The Brookings Institute. 1975.

Alan Soble. "Deception in Social Science Research. Is Informed Consent Possible?" *The Hastings Center Report,* October 1978, p. 40.

The Journal *IRB: A Review of Human Subjects Research,* available through The Hastings Center, focuses explicitly on ethical dilemmas in research on human subjects.

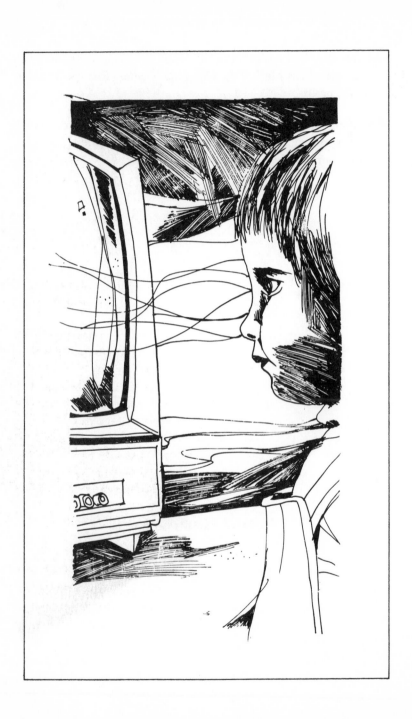

Chapter Eleven

BEHAVIOR MODIFICATION

Introduction

Behavior modification has had a controversial history. Most Americans learned of it as brainwashing. This term was applied to the techniques used to coerce American soldiers to denounce America and its participation in the Korean police action. Similar techniques were popular during the Great Leap Forward and the Cultural Revolution during Mao's attempts to reshape the face of China.

In the United States, Americans were treated to photos of Dr. Delgado of Yale facing a charging bull, protected only by a small box that sent electrical stimuli to the bull's brain. The stimulus stopped the bull in its tracks instantaneously. Human applications were suggested and some individuals had electrodes implanted so that moods could be controlled.

The movies *A Clockwork Orange* and *One Flew Over the Cuckoo's Nest* dramatically illustrated the effects of conditioning programs and the impact of institutions on an individual's ability to shape and change behavior. The message seemed to be that freedom and autonomy were rather fragile and that the reality of rugged individualism may have passed away with other traditional values.

Not all was negative, though. Behavioral programs enabled many individuals with varying degrees of mental retardation to become more self-sufficient, to hold down a job, and to live in a halfway house. Behavior modification helped these individuals achieve a degree of financial and social independence hitherto unthought of.

Other, less dramatic forms of behavior modification are found everywhere. The normal socialization that parents use in raising children is a perfect example. We seldom think of routine activities such as toilet training, learning table manners, dressing oneself, and participating in household chores as forms of behavior modification—but they are.

Another powerful form of behavior modification is education, both formal and informal. Again, as parents realize, when children leave the home other institutions begin shaping behavior. Where the institution is school or a peer group, values and behavior are modified. Current debates over whether and which values should be taught in public schools are as much debates about the power of institutions as they are about the appropriateness of certain values.

Finally, advertising is probably the most universal and perhaps the most effective form of behavior modification. The whole point of advertising is to make you think you need or want what the sponsor wants you to need or want. Much research into the effect of color, shape, environment, and sex appeal of the product or its packaging is done so that the most effective presentation can be made.

In all of these ways—both dramatic and mundane—our behavior is being modified to greater or lesser degrees. In the remaining sections of this chapter, we will look more specifically at some of the techniques of behavior modification and the ethical problems raised by it.

The Techniques of Behavior Modification

Perry London's book *Behavior Control*[1] presented a definition and division of behavior modification that remains helpful in approaching the topic.

Definition

Behavior modification, in London's opinion, is simply defined: changing a person's behavior from one form to another or having that person act the way someone else wants him or her to act. Thus the issue is the fact of a person's behavior changing, not the means whereby this is done. Obviously the means are important and raise ethical questions. But the precise ethical issue of behavior modification is the changing of another person's behavior.

Control by information

The purpose of control through information is ultimately to have the individual gain or regain his or her own independence. Thus even though such control may be initiated or implemented by others, as in psychotherapy, the goal is autonomy, not heteronomy.

The first type of control by information is insight therapy. This is the traditional psychoanalytic model in which the therapist sets a context in which the patient can recall, examine or confront those problems, fears or phobias that prevent him or her from experiencing self-control. This method is more introspective and the patient is responsible for achieving independence.

In action therapy, the second method, the therapist is active and selects methods of therapy or programs to at least relieve the symptoms of the problem so that the patient can regain functional autonomy. While the purpose is still self-control, the therapist is more active in initiating the processes by which that can occur.

Finally, there is conditioning. Here one is trained to respond in a particular way by reacting to a set of simple or complicated signals. This response is then reinforced in some fashion so that a new behavioral pattern is established. The training of animals, the use of biofeedback technologies, and natural childbirth training all employ conditioning to some extent.

Control by coercion

In control by coercion, the subject or patient is almost totally passive. And while self-control is not ignored, control by others is more common in this orientation.

Shock treatment, the first form of control by coercion, can be administered either electrically or chemically. Individuals were induced into a coma by administering insulin in the expectation that this would help schizophrenics achieve control over their personality disorder. Electroconvulsive therapy introduces an electrical current through the brain which produces unconsciousness, temporary memory loss, convulsions, and temporal disorientation. The purpose of this was to relieve anxiety and to help the person achieve self-control.

Second, drug therapy used tranquilizers, sedatives, antidepressants, and psychotropic drugs to control moods and alter perceptions. Many of these drugs effected a genuine breakthrough in the treatment of mentally ill people. These individuals can now live normal lives outside of institutions. Individuals who must remain institutionalized have also benefited, for they no longer need be physically restrained or confined to their ward or room. While one can argue, correctly, that a chemical restraint is still a restraint, nonetheless the degree of freedom provided by these drugs goes a long way in restoring some dignity and freedom to individuals in institutions.

Finally, there is control through the physical invasion of the brain by either surgical procedures or the implantation of electrodes. While the lobotomy is not as popular an operation as it once was, other surgical procedures have proved effective in relieving symptoms and giving relief to patients. The major limitations are the apparent irreversibility of surgical procedures on the brain and the lack of knowledge of what part of the brain controls which specific behavior or symptom. The use of electrodes is physically less problematic because they can be adjusted or removed and they can be controlled more precisely. Also the patient can have a greater degree of autonomy by determining when to send a signal to his or her brain.

Ethical Dilemmas of Behavior Modification

Paternalism

Paternalism is essentially doing something for someone even though he or she has not asked you to do this. In behavior modification, for whose benefit or at whose request is an individual's behavior being changed? And on the basis of whose values will such changes be made?

The applicability of such questions ranges from the evaluation of child rearing practices, the curriculum in a school system, the treatment of patients in hospitals, therapy provided on behalf of the involuntarily institutionalized in mental hospitals, and the current debate about deprogramming former cult members.

In all of these instances individuals are being taught to act in a particular way because it is good for them, because of social expectations, because of the good of society, or because of the superiority of one set of values over another. In all these cases, something is being done to someone when he or she hasn't requested it.

In the previous discussion of paternalism in Chapter 3, I mentioned a process by which paternalistic acts could be evaluated. That process should be referred to now to help evaluate the moral legitimacy of these forms of behavior modification.

Freedom

The reality of freedom, on which informed consent and autonomy are based, is complex in and of itself. In discussions of behavior modification, the complexity of these issues increases geometrically. This is so, first, because the organ which is certainly the sine qua non of our exercising freedom—the brain—is precisely the organ whose capacities are either in question or are damaged. Willard Gaylin of the Hastings Center noted this elementary fact years ago and it has continued to complicate the issues.

Second, how does one understand freedom? Is one free only when one acts without limits, without reasons, without constraints? Or is freedom compatible with institutional pressures, physical and psychological limits, some coercion and/or manipulation?

Paradoxically, many of the forms of behavior modification restrict freedom of choice and freedom of movement only so that these freedoms can be restored to the individual. Thus freedom is established through restrictions.

How one defines freedom and evaluates the relation of means to ends greatly shapes the moral evaluation of the techniques of behavior modification.

Third, obtaining informed consent is obviously problematic. If persons are incapacitated either by illness or by physical harm, they cannot consent for themselves and others must consent for those individuals. This raises issues of paternalism, nonmaleficence, and beneficence. The ethical tension is one of helping the patient as best as one can, while recognizing that the patient cannot be part of the consent process.

Labeling

Giving labels to identify or classify people and their behavior is such a commonplace practice that we seldom think of it as having ethical significance. Almost everybody at some time has had a nickname; we frequently refer to people as yuppies, creeps, or other endearing classifications. Name calling seems to have an honored place in the American way of life.

Labeling or naming does raise moral issues, however. Consider the effect, for example, of identifying someone as crazy, a cult member, or a homosexual. Something much more profound than classification has occurred, for labels such as these carry a moral agenda with them. Labeling individuals as being in the latter categories frequently serves as the basis for discriminatory behavior, the curtailment of civil rights, and attempts to change the individual's values.

Labeling or identifying persons as deviant implicitly suggests that their values or basis of self-identification are not as good as others and are, perhaps, morally inferior or wrong. This ethical evaluation of the basis of identity determines how a person will be treated and what rights will be accorded him or her.

Thus our and society's notions of what is normal, natural, or appropriate serve as the basis of moral evaluation, judgments about sanity, and acceptability. Such value judgments frequently show up in our theories and methods of education, our definitions of mental health, sexual stereotyping, role assignments, and participation in religion. Such a widely accepted but uncritically evaluated concept of normal can serve as the basis for the modification of an individual's behavior. Having labeled someone as a such-and-such, one can then use the right values to correct his or her deviant behavior.

Conclusion

Behavior modification is an exceptionally complex issue. We know the tremendous liberation that individuals have experienced as a result of undergoing various training programs. But we also know the subtle, and frequently unconscious, value judgments that serve as the basis for changing someone's behavior. And we constantly receive any number of stimuli through advertising and the media designed to change our behavior.

And our reactions vary. We may view advertising as obnoxious or delightful, but not as inherently dangerous. Deprogramming cult members is viewed as an attempt to reinsert values allegedly removed by the brainwashing techniques of the cult. Seldom is the cult member asked (or believed) about his or her views. Shock therapy is recognized as dangerous, but coerced repetitions of behaviors are understood to be part of training programs.

Yet, recognizing that there is a reality such as behavior

modification and that we and the institutions of society engage in it frequently helps us to be aware of the issue and more sensitive to the moral issues involved.

Note

1. Perry London, *Behavior Control*. New American Library, 1971, pp. 43ff.

Topics for Discussion

1. Do you think your experience at school has been more indoctrination or education?

2. Do you think cult members should be deprogrammed? Do you think they were brainwashed in the first place?

3. Do you agree with the use of behavior modification techniques to train the mentally retarded?

4. What do you think are the consequences of labeling someone as mentally ill?

5. Are there limits to what mental health professionals can do to cure someone?

Bibliography

A. Bandura, *Principles of Behavior Modification*. Holt, Rinehart, and Winston, 1969.

Jose Delgado, *Physical Control of the Mind: Toward a Psycho-Civilized Society*. Harper and Row, 1969.

Erving Goffman, *Asylums*. Anchor Books, 1961.

Seymour Halleck, *The Politics of Therapy*. Jason Aranson, 1971.

Robert Jay Lifton, *Thought Reform in the Psychology of Totalism. A Study of "Brain Washing" in China*. W.W. Norton and Company, 1969.

Perry London, *Behavior Control*. The New American Library, 1977, Second Edition.

Ruth Macklin, *Man, Mind and Morality. The Ethics of Behavior Control.* Prentice-Hall, 1982.

B. F. Skinner, *Beyond Freedom and Dignity.* Alfred A. Knopf, 1972.

Thomas S. Szasz, *Law, Liberty and Psychiatry. An Inquiry into the Social Uses of Mental Health Practices.* Macmillan, 1963.

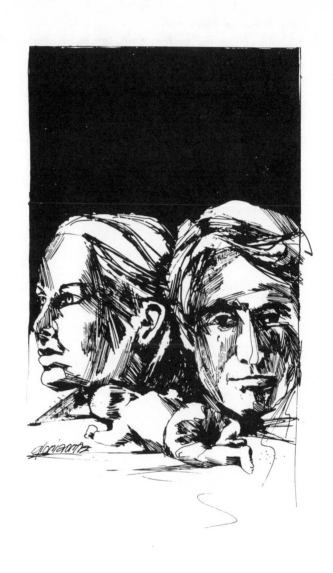

Chapter Twelve

GENETIC ENGINEERING

Introduction

To get a practical idea of how far we have come in the science of genetics and applications through genetic technologies, read or reread *Brave New World* by Aldous Huxley.

This book was written in 1932. At that time, the genetic code had not been discovered (1953), the technology of recombinant DNA research had not been thought of (1970s), external fertilization of a human egg had not been attempted (1978), new life forms had not been invented or patterned (1980), and the transplantation of genes to correct genetic defects had not been attempted (1985).

Yet all of these realities are either assumed or used in the book—in addition to some others currently being worked on in the laboratory. One can regard—and perhaps dismiss—the book as a particularly lucky—though inspired—guess about future technological developments. On the other hand, the book clearly shows how far and how rapidly one can go when the critical insight is reached. Absent the aspects of mass production, the ability to get ninety individuals out of a single egg, a few other manufacturing details, and the socio-political system, we do almost everything Huxley describes.

Along with these new and tremendous powers has come a new attitude toward science. Traditionally, scientists studied natural phenomena to understand them, to be able to formulate the laws that stood behind reality. Thus the major purpose of science was to *describe* nature. Scientists achieved their primary purpose when they were able to formulate basic laws that described how nature operated.

Two events changed that attitude, although such a change was not their primary purpose. The first event was the applied research in many fields that led to the building and detonation of the first atomic bomb. Here the intent was not to discover and describe the laws of nature. The intent was to discover, describe, and *use* the laws of nature. This marks a shift from basic research to applied research. The second event was the discovery of the structure of DNA by Watson and Crick in 1953. This discovery opened the door to significant developments in genetics which culminated in the capacity to recombine genetic material from one organism into another and make a new entity, for example, a bacterium that eats oil, designed to clean up oil spills. These discoveries gave humans the capacity to *change* nature.

We have now—housed under the general heading of genetic engineering—a large number of capacities that enable us to intervene directly into human life—as well as other aspects of nature—and change it according to our designs and wishes. While the ethical justification for such interventions raises several ethical issues, the capacity to redesign humans raises many more.

The purpose of this chapter is to identify and discuss several of the thematic ethical questions raised by the new genetic technologies. While such identification of issues can fall back on traditional philosophical and theological discussions, events continue to outdistance our capacity to even comprehend—let alone evaluate—what is occurring in the rapidly growing field of genetic engineering.

Ethical Issues

General Perspectives

(1) Models of Nature

A background issue that influences many of our discussions of genetic engineering is our understanding of nature or our perceptions of what we can do with it. In an early article, Daniel Callahan identified three basic orientations that influence how we discuss the possibilities of nature.[1]

First, there is the model of nature as plastic. In this perspective, nature is seen as alien and removed from humans. It is plastic in that it can be shaped and used in any way humans see fit. The model assumes that the only limit to nature is the limit humans put on it. Thus, nature is at the disposal of humans.

Second, nature can be experienced as sacred. This tradition finds a home in both Eastern and Western religious traditions. Taoism suggests conformity to nature so that individuals may become part of the cosmic whole of which nature is a manifestation. The medieval theologian Bonaventure, following the lead of Francis of Assisi, saw nature as the footprints of God. The natural was a reflection of the glory of God. These perspectives create an attitude of stewardship or conservation of nature. While one may intervene, such acts should be discreet and infrequent.

Third, we have a teleological model of nature. This understanding suggests that there is a purpose and logic in nature. There is an inner dynamism that leads nature to certain ends or goals. Any interventions must be respectful of these ends. They set a limit which prevents the violation of nature. Thus the extent of interventions into nature is set by the dynamism of nature itself.

What we do is, in part, determined by what we think we can do. If, for example, we think that nature is only an object existing apart from us, we may be willing to consider more interventions than if we thought of it as being part of an organic whole which is sensitive to interventions.

Ironically, the Judaeo-Christian tradition is partly responsible for the desanctification of nature. In its clear and firm rejection of idolatry and its affirmation of God's being a God *of* nature rather than a God *in* nature, tradition validated the objectification of nature. While many in that tradition would not want to intervene to the same extent that others have, nonetheless the balance is a difficult one to maintain.

(2) Responsibilities of the scientist

One of the thematic debates in professional ethics is over the responsibility of the scientist or, speaking more generally, the expert. James Gustafson has proposed several models we can use to work our way through this issue of professional responsibility.[2] These models can help us test different understandings of responsibility and evaluate different consequences of a particular position.

First, scientists have the right to do whatever is possible. The justification for this position is the inherent value of knowledge itself. This is complemented by the valuing of intellectual curiosity and the seemingly inherent human drive to solve problems. In this model, the only limit is the lack of technical capacity.

Second, scientists have no right to intervene in nature. Such a stringent prohibition is based either on a view of nature as sacred or because the proposed research violates a limit imposed by nature. This model is reminiscent of the position of some American Indians who refused to practice agriculture because to do so was to rip up the breast of their mother, the earth. Total consistency in this position would lead to reduction of the human community to hunting and gathering societies. Thus, many individuals would not use this principle absolutely, but understand it, rather, as a strong check on the previous understanding of responsibility.

Third, scientists have no right to change the most distinctive human characteristics. This model of responsibility, related to nature as teleological, sees interventions checked by a particular limit: human characteristics. Thus one can intervene in nature, as opposed to the second model, but human nature is the boundary, not lack of technical capacity, as in the second model.

Finally, scientists have the right to foster the growth of valued human characteristics and to remove those which are harmful. This model suggests a high level of intervention both to control and direct human development. The goal is quality of life. This goal is served by directing human growth and removing obstacles to its fulfillment.

Clearly, none of these are practiced in a pure form but we do find traces of them in most of us. The issue is to use them to help us better understand what we are doing and how we justify it.

(3) Interventionist strategies

The first interventionist strategy is therapeutic. This is a traditional goal within medicine and has as its intent curing or relieving symptoms. Such a therapeutic intent is behind the guidelines on gene therapy, released in September 1985 by the National Institute of Health. These guidelines permit the introduction of a gene into the human body to correct a genetic defect. Although a new procedure, the intent falls within the traditional practice of medicine: healing the sick.

The other interventionist strategy is eugenic, which means well born. The purpose of such an intervention is to improve an organism in some fashion. There are three basic mechanisms for doing this.

1. Positive eugenics. This introduces improvements through selective breeding. Such practices have been performed in animals for centuries. These methods are also being used on humans. The Nobel Prize winners' sperm bank offers the hope of producing very intelligent individuals through the use of sperm from very intelligent men.

2. Negative eugenics. This method keeps bad or inferior genes from entering the gene pool. This can be done by screening parents and informing them of any defective genes they may

carry. It can also be done by amniocentesis. Both methods seek to prevent defective genes from being expressed in an individual so they can be passed on again.

3. Euthenics. This is a modification of the environment so that an individual with a genetic defect can develop relatively normally. Examples of this are eyeglasses to correct myopia, insulin, kidney dialysis machines, and various life support systems.

These three strategies aim at influencing the individual or the environment. The minimal hope is a healthier individual. The maximal hope is a genetically enhanced individual with superior capacities and abilities.

Specific Ethical Issues

(1) Are any and all eugenic interventions acceptable?

Clearly, we are comfortable with the tradition of healing or relief of symptoms. Will we or should we be as comfortable with attempts to optimize human life? Few would dispute the desirability of enhancing the quality of life. Few would dispute preventing a disease from afflicting an individual. Some, however, may dispute attempting to breed only geniuses or scientists or whatever individual trait one may desire. Control over genetic inheritence is a worthwhile enterprise. But as in so many cases, the problem is to what extent we use that power.

(2) What criteria should be used for intervention?

Many criteria for intervention are present: behavioral, social, medical, political, and economic. Each criterion presents a strategy for intervention that reveals a value preference or a priority of values. The how of intervention shows what a society thinks is important and what it will pay to get there. These value choices reveal a picture of human nature, the basis of social organization, and an image of the good of society. The strategies we use to achieve these goals reveal much about our ethical standards.

(3) Who chooses the criteria?

Assuming that interventions are possible, and that criteria can be developed, the critical question remains: Who decides what to do? Some candidates are: scientists, politicians, physicians, citizens, patients, or committees. In selecting a decision-maker, one needs to be aware of the fallacy of the generalization of expertise. This fallacy suggests that since a person is an expert in one area, he or she is also an expert in some or all fields. Obviously expertise is important in decision-making, but we need to be clear about whether we want technical knowledge to be the only relevant factor.

(4) What are the risks of intervention?

Risks can be thought of on an individual, social and, environmental scale. With respect to the individual, the outcome of a particular intervention may not be clear, or there may be risks in achieving the goal. For society, the genetic interventions may begin the process of developing a select type of society or a society in which only a particular segment receives the benefits of genetic intervention. From an environmental perspective, we now have an historical consciousness that reminds us that even the most innocent interventions may have dramatic impacts. Improvements in the quality of grains have led to an increase in bushels per acre and a decrease in price, which is in part responsible for the contemporary American farm crisis. Thus interventions have outcomes that occur in strange and distant places. Thoughtfulness and careful planning must precede any such genetic intervention.

(5) Who receives the benefits?

Genetic interventions have clearly benefited millions of people. We all eat better, live longer, and have more capacities for intervention because of developments in genetics. Yet, how do we know that what we are doing will actually be beneficial, and for whom? A benefit in one area can turn into a burden elsewhere. Euthenic interventions which eliminate childhood diseases allow children to live longer. Yet more children may disrupt the family by straining its resources, disrupting inheritance patterns, especially with respect to land, and causing economic and social problems in the larger society because of the larger population. Again, care must be taken in defining benefits and targeting a recipient population lest one person's benefits become another's burdens.

Areas of Application

Recombinant DNA Research

In this exciting field of research, in which strands of DNA are cut up at various sites, separated, and recombined with other pieces of DNA to create new genetic packages or new entities, there has been much debate as well as many advances. Human insulin has been able to be reproduced this way, a bacterium that eats oil has been developed, and a frost resistant grain has been developed. Yet many problems have been raised.

First was the issue of safety. Concern was raised about a redesigned organism escaping into the environment and causing harm. Thus the security of research facilities and the organism under discussion were debated. Guidelines were established which specify where and under what conditions research can be done.

Second, who is to make decisions about the technology? Originally much of the research was funded publicly through government grants. That gave some degree of regulation to the granting agency through the peer review process. But now many private industries are using this technology and there is no analogous check on the private sector. Thus the issue of control becomes critical, especially when one considers some of the dangerous or harmful ways to which the technology could be put, e.g., germ warfare.

Third, many are concerned about the environmental impact of introducing new organisms into the environment. The concern here is whether the balance of nature might be upset. Could a newly engineered organism cause a disruption that would have ecological consequences? How do we know that the only consequences of introducing a new organism into the environment would be the ones we want? The last few decades have given us a heightened sense of ecological sensitivity, and this is the basis of these concerns.

Committees have been established, regulations developed, and organisms tested and developed. Thus far the record is good. The safety requirements have proved effective and the regulations have not stopped research.

Birth Technologies

Although, strictly speaking, the birth technologies do not involve genetic engineering techniques, they are the technologies most closely associated with genetic engineering in the public's mind. Birth technologies are discussed here because they provide the means whereby other technologies can be applied to the externally conceived human fetus.

The breakthrough technology was the process of in vitro fertilization (IVF). This allows an egg to be fertilized outside the uterus, developed until about eight cell divisions have occurred, and then implanted into a prepared uterus. Once IVF was established as a successful technique, the door was open to all sorts of possibilities.

For example, egg and sperm could come from two unmarried individuals, and the fertilized egg be given to a third person who then gives the baby to yet another couple. Or the egg could come from a donor, the sperm from the husband, the fertilized egg implanted into his wife, and they bear a child with a genetic relation to the husband of the couple. The possibilities are limited only by technical capacity and one's imagination.

Although the technology has been greeted with great acclaim, some problems have been noted, especially by the recent Vatican statement on the ethics of artificial reproduction. While many will disagree with the theological foundation of the document, many more will agree with its concerns and warnings about the uncritical use of these technologies. For example, the technology of IVF is not a cure for a disease. It is a solution to the problem of childlessness. Someone who was infertile before remains infertile after. This raises the issue of the purpose of medicine. Is it to cure a disease or to satisfy wishes?

Second, does this technology implicitly get involved in the business of selling babies, particularly when a surrogate mother is involved? This is a particularly troublesome question and desperately needs clarification.

Third, can the renting or selling of something so intimate to oneself—the uterus—cause one to become alienated from her body. Can it cause the woman to be seen simply as an incubator?

Finally, another technological intervention causes other problems. Usually several eggs are fertilized at once. What does one do with the spare fertilized eggs? The solution now is to freeze them. This then raises the question of ownership or disposal rights, especially in the event that couple die and the fertilized egg becomes orphaned.

The new birth technologies raise many questions. One has the growing sense that it would be good to follow the model of recombinant DNA and have a moratorium of practice until some of the problems are better resolved.

Notes

1. Daniel Callahan, "Living with the New Biology," *The Center Magazine* 4 (July/August, 1972) 4.

2. James Gustafson, "Basic Ethical Issues in the Biomedical Fields," *Soundings* 53 (Summer 1970) 151ff.

Discussion Questions

1. Do you think there are limits to our interventions into nature?

2. Where would you place limits and why?

3. Who do you think should be the decision-maker for the new genetic technologies: scientists, physicians, politicians, the public, the individual?

4. Do you think research could be stopped?

5. If you could, would you be a surrogate mother for someone else? Would you expect to be paid for your services?

Bibliography

Lori Andrews, *New Conceptions*. Ballantine Books, 1985.

Rita Arditti, Renate Duelli Klein, and Shelley Minden, Editors, *Test Tube Women*. Pandora Press, 1984.

Joseph Fletcher, *The Ethics of Genetic Control*. Anchor Books, 1974.

Margo J. Fromer, *Ethical Issues in Sexuality and Reproduction*. The C. V. Mosby Co., 1983.

June Goodfield, *Playing God: Genetic Engineering and the Manipulation of Life*. Random House, 1977.

Clifford Grobstein, "Regulations and Basic Research: Implications of Recombinant DNA." 51 *Southern California Law Review* (1978) 1199.

Leon R. Kass, *Toward a More Natural Science: Biology and Human Affairs*. The Free Press, 1985.

Noel P. Keane and Dennis L. Breo, *The Surrogate Mother*. Everest House, 1981.

Daniel J. Kelves, *In the Name of Eugenics*. Alfred Knopf, 1985.

Marc Lappe, *Genetic Politics: The Limits of Biological Control*. Simon and Schuster, 1979.

President's Commission for the Study of Ethical Problems in Medicine and Biomedical and Behavioral Research, *Splicing Life*. U.S. Government Printing Office, 1982.

Paul Ramsey, *Fabricated Man*. Yale University Press, 1970.

Jeremy Rifkin, *Algeny*. Penguin Books, 1983.

Nicholas Wade, *The Ultimate Experiment*. Walker and Company, 1977.

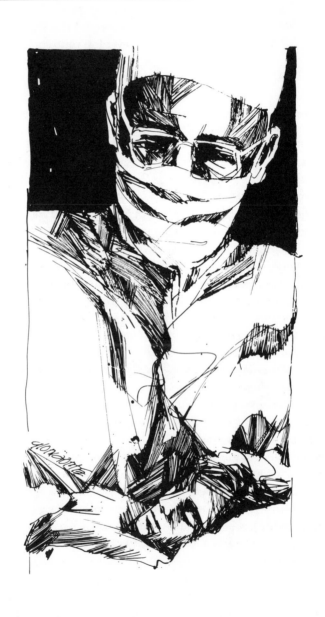

Chapter Thirteen

PATIENTS' RIGHTS

Introduction

Throughout this book we have used the term "rights" frequently. Often the context was that the patient had a right to something. And if we listen to our conversations closely, we will hear ourselves frequently use the term "rights." The word "rights" is almost in danger of losing its meaning and power because of overuse.

And we know that right movements are proliferating. There is an abortion rights movement, civil rights movement, women's rights movement, gay rights movement, animal rights movement, and children's rights movement. No wonder then that when someone hears of a patient's rights movement, the tendency is to dismiss it as "just another one of those movements."

The danger in this is that we forget the place of moral and legal rights within our political and social communities. As in all other areas of life, the abuse or overuse of a concept does not render that concept meaningless. We need to keep in mind the long and difficult social, political and ethical battles that gave us the rights we now take for granted.

The concept of patients' rights is one whose time has come. Historically patients have been assigned a passive role in their treatment. Frequently they were told little, if anything, about what was going on. Sometimes they were not informed about their diagnosis or various treatment options. The motivation for this was not malevolent. Such concealment was seen as a way of protecting the patient, a way of doing no harm. Why add the burden of such information to someone already depressed and worn down by disease.

This practice is slowly reversing itself. Reports of new drugs and treatments are given wider media exposure. Consumers are becoming less afraid of experts. We recognize that expertise has its limits. Many have accepted the practical philosophy that an informed patient is a more cooperative patient. More people are assuming responsibility for their health through various programs of prevention. And, finally, there have been a number of lawsuits which have forced changes in the process of informing patients of their diagnosis and prognosis.

Let us look more closely at the rights movement in medicine by examining the concept of rights, what kinds of rights are being exercised, and what this might mean for the practice of medicine.

Moral and Legal Rights

Moral rights

The social ethics tradition shows two fundamental orientations to rights. The traditional orientation sees rights as a set of mutually binding obligations upon members of a community which allows them to achieve their personal good while simultaneously achieving the common good of the society. Rights arise from membership in the community and tie one to the community. Rights define one's relation to the community, and, through this relationship, one receives certain entitlements.

A more contemporary view sees rights as entitlements to individual goods which the community may not take away. Here rights are defenses against the society. They stake out a zone of privacy around individuals so that they may seek out their best interest. Rights, in this perspective, carry no or only few corresponding duties. The assumption is that society functions best when each pursues his or her own interests.

Legal rights
In both the traditional and contemporary perspective on rights, the focus is on the ethical justification for a certain entitlement or mode of acting. Such an ethical argument, however, confers a claim in law.

Legal rights are those claims to whose fulfillment I am entitled by law. These are rights that are written into law by the community. They specify what claims I may press; they tell exactly and precisely to what I am entitled. Thus legal rights, no matter what their derivation or basis, specify my claims on society, tell what society owes me, and define what limitations, if any, there may be on my rights.

Summary
Not all moral rights are legal rights. Many of the ethical rights we take for granted—freedom of speech, privacy, immunity from self-incrimination, freedom to travel, freedom of religion—were established as legal rights and enshrined in our constitution only after a protracted political and revolutionary struggle.

Some social process is typically necessary to establish a moral or legal right. We should not be surprised that such is also the case in medicine.

The Rights of Patients

The development of the field of health care ethics and the pursuit of several rights in the courts have helped specify many rights in health care. Also the American Hospital Association and the American Civil Liberties Union have developed rights' statements.[1] Finally, federal regulations have specified some rights related to treatment and research. While many of these have been noted and discussed in previous chapters, let me mention some of these rights by way of review and summary.

a. *The right to information.* Probably the most critical right is the one to information. If one is ignorant, one cannot exercise options, cannot make plans, cannot assume control. Access to and possession of information are the bases for exercising autonomy, and if the patient is denied these, he or she will remain a victim of paternalism.

b. *The right to refuse treatment.* If one has the right to give informed consent to treatment, by implication one has the right to refuse treatment. Again such a refusal is an exercise of autonomy and a means whereby the patient exercises the right of self-determination. This right has received strong legal and ethical support. However, it is the right which causes the most difficulties. Health care professionals find it difficult not to help someone. Families may not understand why a member may not want a particular treatment. Society may not accept a particular religion's position on medicine. Thus the good of the individual and the good of society frequently stand in tension.

c. *The right to privacy.* Confidentiality and the protection of information gained during the professional-client interchange are extremely important. If confidentiality cannot be assured, people may not seek help, the basis of a trusting relationship may be destroyed, and a patient's position in society may be jeopardized. Such issues frequently arise in teaching hospitals where many individuals are privy to cases, they arise because health care professionals need to discuss cases with each other, and they arise because records are desired to be examined as part of a research protocol. The recent impetus to identify publicly AIDS victims raises serious privacy and confidentiality issues.

d. *Hospital records.* Two problems frequently present themselves: Can a patient see his or her record, and who, besides the hospital or physician, has access to the record? Frequently patients were not allowed to see their record. This was part of the more general practice of providing little information to the patient. In addition the record contained technical information that the patient might be unlikely to understand. As the right to consent gained more acceptance, so did the right to access to one's records. Again the argument is that one cannot exercise autonomy if one does not have knowledge. The problem of who else can see records is a complex one. The Food and Drug Administration and pharmaceutical companies have an interest in seeing records to understand how new drugs work. Researchers want to examine records to understand disease patterns, causes of diseases, and differences between populations. Insurance companies want to know their clients' health status. The problem of confidentiality is a serious one, especially when there are valid, competing public interest reasons for disclosure.

e. *Voluntary participation in research*. This area is the one in which the most protection of rights is expressed. There is ample ethical argumentation, legal precedent, federal regulation, and institutional support to ensure that potential subjects are recruited and adequately informed before being enrolled in a research protocol. The primary issue here is the protection of the subject. The right of consent is seen as median between the social desire to protect individuals and the needs of science to discover cures for diseases.

Summary

To some, the patients' rights movement may seem like an anti-medicine or anti-physician movement. To some extent this may be correct. Many resent the status and privileges of physicians. Many harbor grudges against physicians. As in all movements, some of the motivation may be misplaced.

But it is also clear that patients have typically been relegated to a passive and/or secondary role. Frequently the patient has been totally left out of the decision-making process. The emphasis on patients' rights seeks to correct this tradition and to ensure that the values and rights of patients occupy their rightful place. This will obviously create problems and cause tension. But as both physician and patient become used to occupying different roles, perceptions and expectations will change and tensions will decrease.

The contribution of the rights movement in medicine has been to place patients within the decision-making process. As in all other areas of life, time is necessary to learn how to exercise these rights, to redefine relationships based on these rights, and to restructure the physician-patient relation. As long as both physicians and patients recognize that the purpose of the discussion of rights is to ensure a better ethical standard in medicine, both can enter into the discussion and practice of rights in medicine as a joint enterprise.

Note

1. For a copy of the AHA's Patient's Bill of Rights, see Martin Benjamin and Joy Curtis, *Ethics in Nursing,* Oxford University Press, 1981. For the ACLU position, see George Annas, *The Rights of Hospital Patients,* Avon Press, 1975.

Discussion Questions

1. What do you think were the main motivations for the development of the patients' rights movement?

2. Do you think the patients' rights movement takes away appropriate responsibility from the physician?

3. Should patients' rights take priority over a physician's medical judgment?

4. Do you think the patients' rights movement will improve or harm the quality of medical care?

5. How should a patient inform a physician that he or she wants an active role in the relationship?

Bibliography

George Annas, *The Rights of Hospital Patients.* Avon Press, 1975.

David Belgum, *When It's Your Turn To Decide.* Augsburg Press, 1978.

Nora K. Bell, *Who Decides? Conflicts of Rights in Health Care.* Humana Press, 1982.

Linda B. Besch, "Informed Consent: A Patient's Right." *Nursing Outlook* 27 (January 1979) 32–35.

Eric Cassell, *The Healer's Art. A New Approach to the Doctor-Patient Relationship.* J. B. Lippincott Company, 1976.

Ruth Macklin, "Rights in Bioethics." In *The Encyclopedia of Bioethics,* Warren Reich, Editor. The Free Press, 1978.

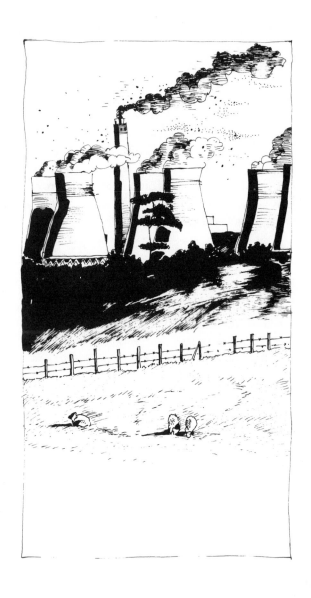

Chapter Fourteen

A WHOLE EARTH ETHIC

Introduction

Hovering at the edges of many of the questions we have discussed are several, broader issues. These issues lead us beyond the physician-patient relation into a wider discussion of problems that are primarily social in nature, even though the individual is involved. Some we have discussed: the allocation of resources emerged repeatedly; our obligations to future generations was involved in the discussion of genetic engineering; social versus individual priorities emerged in the discussion of research.

The reason for titling this chapter as I did is that the problems to be discussed here need to be addressed from the perspective of the whole earth. The concerns and implications of the problems are that great. And while some of these problems may also have an individual dimension—for all ethical concerns ultimately descend upon the individual—the impact of individual actions has profound and long-lasting results.

These problems are important to consider, in a preliminary fashion, to round off our discussion of the other bioethical problems discussed in this book. The rest of this chapter will describe several of these problems and then provide a summary.

The Problems of a Whole Earth Ethic

Population

If there is one thing that is true about the human species, it is not an endangered species. We have so successfully reproduced that ours is the opposite problem: overpopulation. While we have not reached the point of licensing space or issuing permits for reproduction, as some commentators predicted would happen, we are in the beginnings of a population crisis.

We know that the population of China is over one billion people. The population of India is rapidly approaching that same number. And Latin American birth rates are increasing. Thus in terms of absolute numbers, the population is increasing dramatically in some parts of the world. And while some countries are responding severely—China—others do not have population control as a major priority.

Several problems need to be considered here. First, and in some ways most importantly, is the issue of perspective. Is Latin America's population growth a problem because it might mean that North America's standard of living might have to change? That is, is the population problem a problem primarily because of the rate of growth or because of the implication of the rate of growth for other world economies? Problems are always problems for someone, and it is important to determine who defines the problem and on what basis.

Second, and related to this problem, is the imposition of values by one nation on another. Many of the developed nations provide funding for population control programs in underdeveloped nations. The problem is that while the developed nation may see population control as a good in itself, such programs may violate a particular culture's social and/or religious values about reproduction or children. Such funding of population programs may simply be another form of imperialism.

Third, there is the tension between an individual's reproductive freedom and the good of a particular society. The right to reproduce is a fairly basic human right and part of the concept of the sanctity of life as defined earlier in this book. Yet there are pressing social needs and resources and, even though distributed fairly, they can stretch only so far. China, for example, has made remarkable strides in solving the malnutrition problems that plagued it for centuries. But now, because of its population growth, famine is again a possibility for China. The reaction has been a stringent population control policy of one child per family. This policy is enforced through advocating marriage at a later age, use of contraceptives, social pressure, negative incentives, and abortion to back up contraceptive failure. Individual Chinese are being asked to reverse one of their deepest cultural values—children—for the social good.

Food

One of the dominant media images of the last decade is that of starving children. While we may have become hardened or grown numb in the face of continual exposure to the problem, still the images of the devastation from famine catch us up short.

This is especially true because we know that there is a surplus of food in the world. We know that grain rots in American storage bins. Annually we read of record harvests, especially in the United States. Yet people die of starvation and of diseases to which individuals have a lower resistance because of malnutrition.

Surplus is the reason why, first, many suggest that the problem is not the adequacy of food supplies, but one of distribution. And distribution is complicated by political relations (or lack thereof) between nations, by fears of control, by imperialism, and by the implications of a nation's failure to provide for its own citizens. Clearly distribution is a major problem.

But, second, so is the quantity. Much of the success of the record harvests in the United States is the result of heavy use of fertilizers. These fertilizers are expensive and require the ability to make high capital investments. Second, the harvests require the mechanization of farming. The traditional family farm will probably not be able to feed population levels in many underdeveloped countries. Third, many of the grains are hybrids, and while they can produce more bushels per acre, these grains are not hardy and are prone to many blights. Thus many of the hopes of the green revolution were dashed when the new grains did not survive well in natural environments.

This issue leads, third, to the relation between food and population. Assuming that the distribution problems have been solved and that there has been a transition to contemporary agriculture methods, the question still remains of whether supply can keep up with demand. A country may be producing as much food as it can and still not be able to keep up with the population growth. There is a vicious circle operating here. The better fed a population is, the lower the infant mortality rate. The lower the infant mortality rate, the more people survive and the larger the population becomes. This then can cause problems of malnutrition if the supply cannot keep up with the population.

Fourth, what does providing food aid do for a country? In the short run, people are fed, starvation is relieved, and consciences are satisfied. But what happens in the long run? Only providing food does not address the underlying problems of the cause of the famine. These may be overpopulation, poor or inadequate agriculture policies, or a consequence of distribution problems.

This position would differentiate between episodic relief because of crop failure due to drought or some other natural disaster and relief which merely prolongs a nation's coming to terms with intrinsic policy problems. Thus some would justify withholding aid to coerce nations into resolving their problems. In this perspective, aid simply prolongs the agony of a nation and allows it to continue its irresponsibility at the expense of those nations who would benefit from such aid while they make the transition to self-sufficiency and responsibility.

Finally, taking the previous point one step further, food can be a weapon of war. In an analogy to the old siege, one nation can attempt to starve another nation into political submission. Here the issue is not promoting self-sufficiency, but conquest. Populations are hostage, not to internal development policies, but to international politics. While death occurs in war, those who die are usually soldiers. Here the victims are whole populations.

The Environment

One of the major shifts in consciousness of the last several decades is the awareness of the inter-connectedness of our environment. This ecological mind-set has emerged, unfortunately, not as a consequence of sensitivity to the environment, but because of the consequences of several centuries of insensitivity to it. Our careless disposal of chemicals, for example, has come back to haunt us through increased levels of cancer and water unfit to drink. Our wasteful consumption habits have caused the near depletion of many nonrenewal resources.

The first issue is land use or conservation. One author has proposed four ways of thinking of this concern.[1]

1. Resource conservation. The purpose of this viewpoint is to curtail the thoughtless exploitation of forests, wildlife, farmland, and so forth. The intent is to preserve nature for the good of the many, rather than for the profit of the few. The prime issue is avoiding the exploitation of the environment.

2. Wilderness preservation. This perspective focuses on preserving the environment for its own sake. In this view, the environment—forests, wilderness areas, rivers, the Grand Canyon—are valuable in and of themselves, regardless of whether or not they are appreciated by humans. Thus nature is a sort of sacred place, a sanctuary that should not be violated.

3. Moral extensionism or natural moralism. This position argues that humans have duties to natural entities, and that the rights on which these duties are founded are based on some intrinsically valuable characteristic of the entity. Thus, dolphins should be protected because they are intelligent. Rain forests are valuable because of their contribution to the ecology. The important feature of this perspective is that it breaks with the tradition of seeing the environment as valuable only because of its relation to humans. The environment has more than instrumental value—it has meaning in and of itself.

4. Ecological sensibility. This orientation involves three orientations. First, respect is owed anything that has an end of its own or some capacity for internal self-regulation. Second, there is an understanding of reality that takes into account the importance of relationships and systems, as well as human beings. Third, there is an ethic that is orientated in the direction of peaceful co-habitation with nature that involves a restrained and respectful use of it.

All of these orientations imply, first, a very respectful attitude toward nature and, second, varying degrees of the permissibility of intervention. To obtain the full import of these attitudes, one should compare them to the models of nature in Chapter 12. One should especially think of nature as a plastic model, for this seems to be the basic attitude operative in Western societies.

The major debate is not over whether one can intervene in nature; the issue is to what extent one can do this. The model of ecological sensibility does not prohibit interventions into nature, but it certainly would severely critique many of the ways we have gone about intervening. While the most liberal of the four models, it still runs contrary to dominant cultural values.

One can evaluate these models more adequately by determining how each would evaluate the following problems: acid rain, hazardous waste disposal sites, the depletion of nonrenewable resources, strip mining, the development of more national and/or state parks, and genetic engineering.

An ethic of the land or an ethic of the responsible use of resources provides an interesting standpoint from which to evaluate many of the problems we have discussed in this book as well as opening the door to different, more national perspectives. The debate about the wise and responsible use of our resources and how they relate to our food and energy needs is an especially important one. Our resolution of that debate determines what world we leave to our descendants.

Animal rights

The animal rights movement is, first, a logical extension of an environmental ethic that is respectful of the environment and its inhabitants. Second, it is a response to the ways in which animals have been used in some experiments. The animal rights movement is not of recent vintage, however. The anti-vivisection movement antedates the animal rights movement and has kept the issue of the irresponsible use of animals in experiments in the public's eye.

There are two basic forms of animal rights orientations. The first is the more strict movement which argues that animals and humans are on the same moral level with respect to how they can be treated. The basis for ascribing rights or at least interests to animals is their capacity to feel pain. This orientation is combined with a rejection of speciesism, the conferring of status on the human species because it has power. These two orientations combine to found an ethic which rejects any human use of animals. And as a sign of their consistency, members of the animal rights movement are typically vegetarians.

The second orientation is more utilitarian in nature. It sees animals as at the disposal of humans but defines the limit of their use in terms of its effect on humans. Here the ethical standard for the treatment of animals is centered on humans. The standard is that humans treat animals in such a way that the humans do not become desensitized to pain or brutalized by their treatment of animals. Thus the ethic focuses, not on the right or interests of animals, but on what effects on humans treating animals in a particular way will have.

One of the characteristics of the animal rights debate, originally in England but now too in the United States, is the growing activism of those in the rights movement. Labs are raided, animals liberated, injunctions issued, and research terminated. Clearly these activities have focused attention on the conditions in which animals are housed in labs, the worthwhileness of the experiments to which they are submitted, and the pain they undergo. As such the movement has been responsible for either initiating higher standards in the labs or being more responsible with respect to the standards in place.

But the second orientation accepts the subjugation of animals to humans, their use in experiments, and their function as a major food source. And while this orientation would seek to accomplish these goals as humanely as possible, pain will continue to be inflicted on animals and they will continue to be eaten. And the use of animals as a source of organs, for transplantation into humans, as was done in the Baby Fae case, raises new and complex issues in this debate.

Summary

This chapter has raised problems that are exceptionally complex. They have to do with the traditional problem of resolving the tension between individual behavior and the common good. But they also raise problems concerning national and international policy. Acid rain, for example, cannot be solved only by one nation. The same is true with respect to resolving energy issues and toxic waste disposal. How we use land and resources says a lot about us, but the issue transcends individual behavior. Each individual can be responsible in terms of conservation, food habits, and waste disposal, but the country as a whole will still generate waste and will still consume resources to generate energy.

The difficulty of the problems does not excuse our not debating them. In fact the difficulty of the problems should motivate us to immediately debate the issues and to seek to resolve them.

Note

1. John Rodman, "Four Forms of Ecological Consciousness Reconsidered." In *Ethics and the Environment,* Donald Scherer and Thomas Attig, Editors. Prentice-Hall, 1983, pp. 82–92.

Discussion Questions

1. Do you think better distribution of food will solve the problems of famine?

2. Do you think we can grow enough food to feed whatever population is present?

3. Do you think overpopulation is a real problem?

4. Do you think individuals can be restricted in their childbearing practices?

5. Which position do you take toward the environment and why?

6. Do you think animals have rights? Do you think they deserve protection and why?

Bibliography

Bruce Ackerman, *The Uncertain Search for Environmental Quality*. The Free Press, 1984.

William Aiken and Hugh LaFollette, Editors, *World Hunger and Moral Obligation*. Prentice-Hall, 1977.

Rachel Carson, *Silent Spring*. Houghton Mifflin, 1962.

Garrett Hardin, *Exploring New Ethics for Survival*. Penguin Books, 1975.

Garrett Hardin and J. Baden, Editors, *Managing the Commons*. W. H. Freeman, 1977.

Aldo Leopold, *A Sand Country Almanac*. Oxford University Press, 1949, reissued in 1981.

Leo Marx, *The Machine in the Garden*. Oxford University Press, 1973.

Tom Regan and Peter Singer, Editors, *Animal Rights and Human Obligations*. Prentice-Hall, 1976.

Peter Singer, *Animal Liberation*. New York Review, 1975.

Christoper Stone, *Should Trees Have Standing?* William Kaufman, 1974.

Susan Toton, *World Hunger*. Orbis Books, 1982.

Lynn White, "The Historical Roots of Our Ecological Crisis." *Science*. 155 (March 10, 1967) 1203–07.

Robert M. Veatch, Editor, *Population Policy and Ethics. The American Experience*. The Irvington Publishing Co., 1977.